S0-ABO-753

REVLON
ART
OF
BEAUTY

Dolphin Books

DOUBLEDAY & COMPANY, INC.

Garden City, New York

THIS BOOK WAS CREATED
BY THE PEOPLE OF REVLON
under the supervision of
Sharon Queeney,
Director of Consumer Information,
and
Cynthia Morris,
a Revlon Writer.

The technical information in this book
was derived from the Revlon Research
Group. This worldwide body of scien-
tists and technicians works within the
highly advanced facilities of the Revlon
Research Center with the guidance of
Earle W. Brauer, M.D., Revlon Vice
President of Medical Affairs.

Library of Congress Cataloging in Publication Data
Main entry under title:

Revlon art of beauty.

   1. Beauty, Personal.   2. Cosmetics.   I. Revlon, inc.
II. Title: Art of beauty.
RA778.R443   646.7'042
ISBN 0-385-17871-9   AACR2
Library of Congress Catalog Card Number 81-43587

This Workbook Was Produced In Soft Cover because the binding permits the pliancy that work pages require. The work pages, 74-79, serve as a canvas for coloring and creating new face looks and provide a medium for experimenting and expressing your makeup ideas.

TO REVLON, beauty is an applied art. It is a language of **color, and of drama and of emotion.** It is a standard of being that reflects the way you live and the way you feel about yourself.

Introduction

If you haven't already done so, it is time to introduce a new facet into your life — the art of beauty. Starting now, you can actually learn to live up to your own beauty potential — to look **more vital, more attractive, more totally fit.**

REVLON ART OF BEAUTY is based on Revlon's philosophy that beauty is individual. To provide you with person-to-person attention, basic beauty techniques in treatment and color are personalized according to different facial characteristics. This individualized guidance should enable you to look your best.

the news is this

No matter how your skin looks today — it can look even better. Proper care is the key. Starting now, what you do for your skin will make a dramatic difference in the way you look tomorrow. The pages that follow offer the information you need to improve the look and feel of your skin.

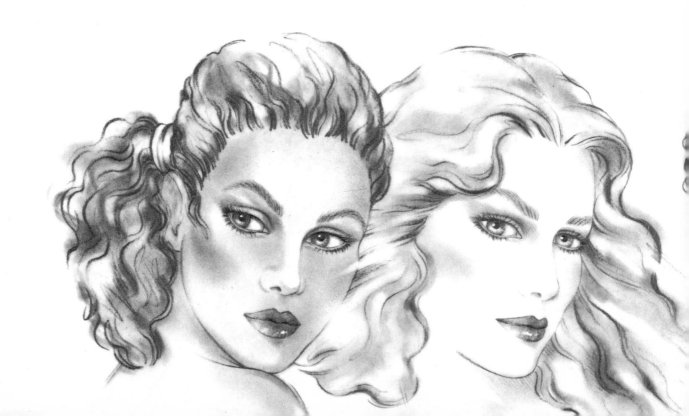

SKIN

A REFLECTION OF THE WAY YOU LIVE AND FEEL

Just about everyone is born with healthy, beautiful skin, but time and neglect give birth to imperfections. **Skin is the body's screening system.** It projects deficiencies in diet, sleep, exercise and skin care. Practicing good living habits has a significant effect on your skin's physical fitness — its resiliency, texture and coloring. Getting the most out of your skin is what beauty treatments are designed to do. There are skin care products perfected to meet **your** skin's specific characteristics and its changing needs.

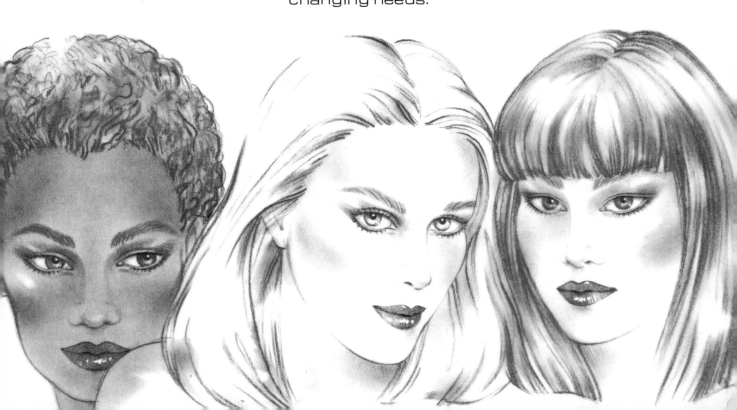

EPIDERMIS

DERMIS

SUB-DERMIS

AMAZINGLY

BEFORE YOU CAN CHART

an effective course of beauty, it's important to understand how your skin functions.

1 The surface (cosmetic) layer of the skin is called the epidermis. This outer layer is where new cells are constantly being formed. By the time these new cells travel 28 days to the surface of your skin, they're depleted of moisture and slough off. The epidermis also contains living cells that produce melanin, the pigment that gives skin and hair their color.

2 The second layer and key section of the skin is called the dermis. The skin's major support system, the dermis contains blood vessels that house your skin's supply of oxygen and also distribute nutrients to the skin. The dermis produces collagen as well, a protein ingredient that helps your skin appear healthy, resilient and youthful.

3 The innermost layer of the skin is referred to as the sub-dermis. This hidden tier of skin contains fatty tissue and muscle.

the epidermis — the visible part of your skin — is only 1/1000 of an inch thick. That means your whole appearance depends on the visible condition of less than a millimeter of skin.

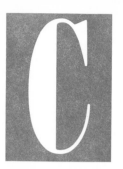 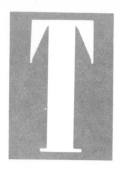 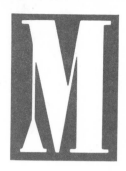

The basics of good skin care are as simple and straightforward as 1, 2, 3. So make them an automatic part of your A.M. and P.M. grooming. Keep these letters on tap in your mind **C T M** because this is your fail-safe beauty formula to follow faithfully, day and night.

WHAT DOES PROPER CLEANSING DO?

CLEANSE

1 Dissolves makeup and removes excess oils, bacteria and dirt that can block pores and gradually develop into blemishes
2 Eliminates the outer layer of dead skin cells that can dull skin
3 Promotes a brighter, fresher appearance

Facial cleansers come in various forms: solid and liquid soaps, lotions and creams designed for the needs of different skin types. It's important to use the correct facial cleanser since it is synchronized to your skin's characteristics.

WHAT DOES PROPER TONING DO?

TONE

1 Removes excess oils and cleanser residue
2 Refines pores for a smoother appearance
3 Stimulates and refreshes the skin
4 Promotes a more youthful radiance
5 Prepares skin to receive the maximum benefits of a moisturizer

After-cleansing products are called Toners, Fresheners and Astringents. These terms are used interchangeably. The mildest forms are free of alcohol and best suited for dry skin. Those that contain alcohol come in various strengths. Ask questions before you buy.

MOISTURIZE

WHAT DOES PROPER MOISTURIZING DO?

1 Replenishes natural moisture loss

2 Minimizes the appearance of dry lines

3 Cushions the effects of harsh weather

4 Provides longer wear for makeup and helps to keep its color fresh-looking

MOISTURE IS THE DIFFERENCE BETWEEN A RAISIN AND A GRAPE

Physically fit skin is almost 90% water. And it's the water-and-oil balance that keeps your skin soft and supple. Moisturizers are offered in both lotions and creams ranging from lightweight and fast-absorbing to rich and emollient. Some formulas are enhanced with special ingredients like soluble collagen.

HOW TO SELECT A MOISTURIZER

The way a moisturizer acts and feels has a lot to do with its capabilities. Massage it into your face.

- Is it the consistency you prefer, i.e., lightweight or creamy?
- Does it absorb quickly into the skin?
- Does it leave a soft glow and a silky finish?

If more moisturizer stays on top of your skin than is absorbed, it is probably richer than your skin needs.

CHECK the square next to the skin type you think you have. Then turn to the skin section that applies to you.

NOW THAT YOU KNOW the fundamentals of proper skin care and the general types of products to use, the next step is to perfect your program — to customize this information to your skin's individual needs. That requires a proper introduction to the three basic skin types. So read the following descriptions for **dry, normal and oily skin.**

☐ **EVIDENT SIGNS OF DRY SKIN**

- A generally tight, taut feeling to skin
- Obvious lines around eyes, mouth or on forehead
- Few problems with skin breakout and blemishes
- Dull, parched or flaky appearance

☐ **NOTICEABLE SIGNS OF NORMAL SKIN**

- Visible pores, basically smooth texture
- Neither primarily dry nor oily
- Somewhat oilier T-Zone (forehead, nose and chin)
- Either monthly breakout or infrequent breakout

☐ **OBVIOUS SIGNS OF OILY SKIN**

- Overall oily shine, particularly on the T-Zone
- Enlarged pores, especially on the cheeks
- Problems with blackheads, whiteheads or acne breakout
- Flakiness around nose and chin (accumulation of dried oils)

TEST

Smile into a mirror. If your face feels tight or if you find laugh lines around your eyes, mouth or on your forehead that aren't funny, and appear before their time, you are clearly a dry skin type.

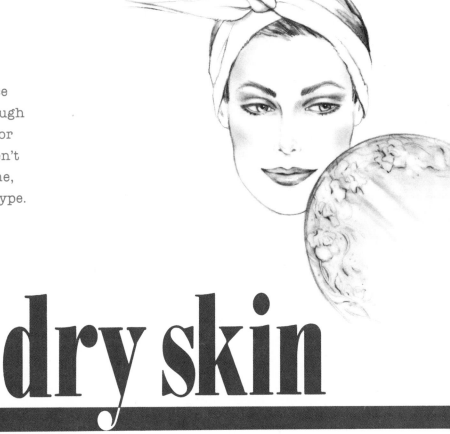

dry skin

Because dry skin is fragile, the signs of aging are more prominent than in other skin types. It chaps easily and is vulnerable to cold and sun. So gentle care and moisture protection products are crucial to its good condition.

Dehydration is your worst enemy. So whatever you do, guard against excessive exposure to air conditioning and central heating — both of which rob skin of moisture. And moisture is what dry skin needs plenty of — because the thinner the skin is, the more difficulty it has retaining moisture. Remember, too, that careful handling in applying and removing beauty creams will help keep your face physically fit.

PROVEN PLAN FOR DRY SKIN

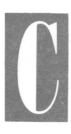

CLEANSING

Gentle and mild are two words you must always consider when choosing a cleanser. Cleanse your face morning and night with a cream, lotion or soap product developed for dry skin (usually a water-rinsable or tissue-off type).

These products are richer formulations that help quench your thirsty skin and leave it soft and smooth. If you decide to use a face soap, select an emollient, dry skin cosmetic soap. Be sure to rinse thoroughly as soap residue can dry skin. Should drying side effects appear, switch to a lotion or cream cleanser.

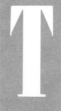

TONING

Be sure your toner or freshener is a gentle formulation for dry skin or one that is free of alcohol. Saturate a cotton ball and gently remove the last traces of cleanser residue. This prepares your skin for moisturizing and helps give your face a fresh radiance.

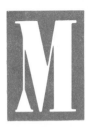 **MOISTURIZING**

DAYTIME MOISTURIZING

This is your skin's most important beauty treatment, so make your choice a good one. Your moisturizer should be rich in emollients. Remember to concentrate on your forehead and the area around your mouth, and to use an eye cream every day.

NIGHTTIME MOISTURIZING

Night cream is a more concentrated form of moisturizer. It is richer by design to give you effective through-the-night moisturizing. Yours should be abundant in lubricants and humectants to produce the results you'll want to see by morning.

So when you buy your moisturizer, be sure to ask for one that contains those ingredients. Don't forget to treat your neck to a protective veil of night cream and to pat on an eye treatment before the lights go out.

WEEKLY MOISTURIZING

A moisturizing masque is your skin's beauty bonus. Most of these masques are composed of proteins and minerals in a lubricating base that help give your skin additional moisture nourishment.

FACE-SAVERS
• Drink at least 8 glasses of water a day • Wear moisturizer 24 hours a day, every day • Apply moisturizer under a moisturizing masque • Use a sunscreen to guard against harsh rays • Use moisturizer before blow-drying your hair • Try not to squint — dry skin is apt to line • Moisturize around eyes and on neck every night

normal skin

Normal skin is actually "combination skin," meaning it is drier on the cheeks and around the hairline and oilier at the center of the face. Don't let your skin's usually problem-free behavior make you lax in your beauty habits.

Maintenance is a must to keep combination skin in top form. And without it, your skin will begin to show signs of neglect and aging long before it should. The right products for you are those designated as normal-to-dry or normal-to-oily.

PROVEN PLAN FOR NORMAL SKIN

CLEANSING

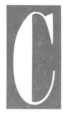

Depending on your skin's tendencies, select either a facial soap or a gentle rinse or tissue-off lotion. Be sure it's the best formulation for you. Cleanse your face morning and night. If you have oily T-Zone shine, boost cleansing benefits by using a soft complexion brush or facecloth on oily area.

T TONING

Use a medium-strength toner twice a day after cleansing your face and a full-strength toner on your oilier T-Zone as often as you think necessary. This toning procedure will help keep your normal/combination skin healthy-looking.

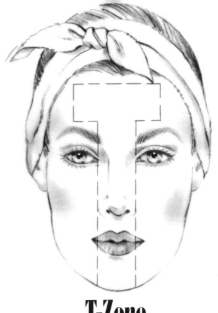

T-Zone

M MOISTURIZING

DAYTIME MOISTURIZING

Lightweight moisturizer is best for normal-to-oily skin. Use richer formulations for normal-to-dry skin. Concentrate application on drier areas and expression lines. Gently pat on eye cream under the eyes from the outer corner toward the nose.

NIGHTTIME MOISTURIZING

Use night cream to help balance the oil/moisture content in your skin. If skin is normal-to-oily, you may find your daytime moisturizer adequate for night. Or, use daytime moisturizer on oilier areas and a richer formula on drier areas as well as your neck. Apply eye cream for overnight care.

WEEKLY FACIAL MASQUES

Select a masque for normal skin — preferably a cleansing masque. Use it once a week if you have normal-to-dry skin or twice weekly if your skin is normal-to-oily. Be sure to apply a moisturizer immediately following its use. During colder months, when skin tends to be drier, you may opt to alternate with a moisturizing masque.

TEST

Take this oil-check test two mornings in a row. Be sure you are not wearing a night treatment the nights before you plan to take this morning test. Upon waking, press a tissue to your face, particularly the T-Zone area. If the tissue is saturated with oil, your skin is clearly oily.

oily skin

The main objective: control shine and oil buildup so skin looks cleaner and makeup wears longer. Use highly concentrated formulations with antiseptic capabilities to reduce your chances of skin eruptions — blackheads, whiteheads, etc. While your skin may not always be on good behavior, oiliness gives it a built-in youth factor since oil helps prevent dry lines.

FOR EXTRA-OILY SHINE, cleanse 3 times a day or, if that's not possible, use a toner during the day to remove excess oil. Then reapply your makeup.

PROVEN PLAN FOR OILY SKIN

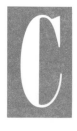

CLEANSING

Oily skin picks up more outdoor grime and pollutants than drier skin so cleanse thoroughly and often. Facial soap formulated for oily skin is your ideal cleanser. Massage lather over your face with a washcloth or soft-bristled face brush to keep excess oil in check and help dislodge blackheads. Another option is a rinse-off lotion made for oily skin.

T TONING

After cleansing, use a toner that contains alcohol so your skin will get the kind of deep-cleansing treatment it needs. Special midday toning will also help curb excess oil and shine.

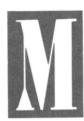

MOISTURIZING

DAYTIME MOISTURIZING

The one thing your skin doesn't need is more shine, so buy a light, water-based moisturizer and apply sparingly. Remember, moisture is not oil, so even oily skin needs the benefits of a moisturizer— particularly drier areas such as the neck and outer portions of the face.

NIGHTTIME MOISTURIZING

Traditional night creams are too rich in lubricants for oily skin. Use your daytime moisturizer at bedtime and, if you are prone to breakout, alternate it with a medicated product.

WEEKLY OIL CHECK

Your skin care program, morning to night to weekly, is based on high-performance cleansing. Apply a cleansing masque at least once a week to minimize excess oil. Clay masques are particularly beneficial since they help tighten pores.

FACE-SAVERS

● Cleanse skin thoroughly—3 times a day ● Use oil-reducing skin care products and an oil-control stick ● Use a toner for on-the-job or on-the-go cleansing ● Use pressed powder to control oil and freshen makeup

19

HIGHLIGHTS ON DARKER SKIN

Everyone's skin contains melanin, which gives skin and hair its color. In darker skin tones, the melanin-producing cells are more active and deposit pigment in the epidermis, which gives the appearance of darker skin.

The melanin in darker skin accounts for the wide and vivid variations of complexion tones. And, oddly enough, the darker your skin tone, the more noticeable scarring from blemishes and skin irritations tends to be.

HERE'S WHAT YOU CAN DO TO HELP:

Use the skin care products and program that are right for you every day to help reduce the likelihood of breakout and keep your skin in better form.

■ Use a tinted moisturizer to help even out skin coloring and a cover stick to minimize dark spots and blotchiness.

■ For freckles, age spots or minor discolorations, use a fade cream containing hydroquinone to gently and gradually lighten these areas.

CAUTION

If skin begins to lighten in spots (hypopigmentation) or becomes seriously darker (hyperpigmentation), be sure to consult a dermatologist.

GET TO KNOW YOUR SKIN
Answer true or false to the following questions:

1 **TRUE OR FALSE:**   Fade creams can be used to lighten and brighten your overall complexion.

2 **TRUE OR FALSE:**   If nothing else is available, a light coating of petroleum jelly is better for dry skin than no moisturizer at all.

3 **TRUE OR FALSE:**   Darker skin does not need sunscreen protection.

ANSWERS

1 **TRUE**   Fade creams will lighten your overall complexion and react on areas where an overproduction of melanin has caused dark spots.

2 **TRUE**   Petroleum jelly is better than nothing at all, but it is not prepared for your delicate beauty needs. Its heavy, greasy consistency lies on the skin's surface and can clog pores. Beauty creams formulated for your facial skin are more effectively absorbed by the skin and also provide a base for makeup application.

3 **FALSE**   Darker skin needs sun protection. While the higher melanin concentration provides darker skin with some solar protection, if you have been sunbathing for any prolonged period you know that your skin can burn too.

SUN SAFETY   The lighter your natural skin coloring, the more sun protection you need. Read labels and choose the Sun Protection Factor (SPF) that is best for you. Numbers range from 2 to 15 and higher. Each number defines the amount of time you can safely stay in the sun. SPF 2 provides 2 times longer protection than you would have without a sunscreen product. SPF 4 offers 4 times longer protection, etc.

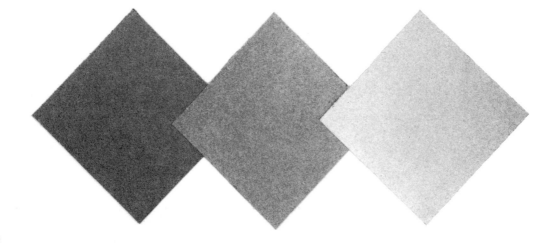

YOUNG SKIN IS IN FULL BLOOM

- High oil-and-moisture content makes skin soft, supple and more resilient.
- The complexion has a vibrant, youthful cast.
- Muscle tone is in peak condition.
- Blood circulates more freely, speeding vitamins and essential nutrients to the skin.

SELF-HELP FOR TEENAGE SKIN

When lipsticks replace lollipops, it's time for good skin care.

If you are already aware of this, you belong at the head of the class. Maintaining the qualities of young skin is what proper skin care is all about. While some teenage skin may be normal-to-dry, more often it tends to be oily. The rate of hormonal activity during adolescence can produce enough excess oil to disturb the skin. The result: breakout or acne. For advice on what you can do to help counteract this problem, refer to these sections of the book:

ACNE-PRONE SKIN, Page 32.

FACE-SAVERS, Page 19.

GET INTO HEALTHY HABITS, Page 26.

When it comes to caring for your skin, **make cleansing the main event.** That doesn't mean that any soap you find in the soap dish is right. Like all skin, teenage skin needs the special benefits of a facial cleanser — keyed to skin type.

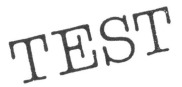

TEST

Pinch the skin on the knuckle of a finger. Release it and notice the sluggish manner in which it falls back into place. This is how skin that has lost its resiliency behaves.

SELF-HELP FOR MATURE SKIN

THE AGING PROCESS:

CAUSE & EFFECT

1 Sebaceous (oil-producing) glands become less productive.

2 Cells retain less moisture and lose their fullness.

3 Normal skin functions slow down.

Although the loss of skin resiliency occurs all over the body, it is most pronounced on the exposed areas — face, neck, hands and arms. <u>Mature skin needs every ounce of moisture it can get.</u> While there is nothing you can do to prevent biological causes of aging skin, you can adopt measures that will greatly reduce the effects of exterior causes.

WHAT AGES AND LINES YOUR SKIN?

● Prolonged sun exposure ● Harsh weather and biting winds ● Your living habits — what you do and eat ● Exaggerated facial expressions ● Lack of proper skin care

ACTION:

Now that you know the causes and effects, here are some self-help measures to put into motion.

1 Try to reduce the use of soaps on your skin (face and body).

2 Choose products that contain moisturizing ingredients and soluble collagen.

3 Make sun-protective products a consistent part of your skin care plan.

4 Avoid sunbathing between the hours of 11 A.M. and 3 P.M. when rays are strongest.

5 Use creams and makeup on cold days to help buffer your face against dryness and skin-freezing temperatures.

6 Once a week, apply a firming masque and follow with a moisturizing masque.

7 Try to avoid exaggerated facial expressions that create unnecessary lines.

"Moisturizing is crucial to maintaining youthful-looking skin. From the age of 35 and on, make certain to concentrate on moisturizing the skin below your collarbone."

FIVE POINTERS FOR EVERYONE

- Drink 6-8 full glasses of water a day.

- Eat with beauty in mind — fresh fruits and vegetables, fewer fats and fried foods.

- Exercise every day to keep fit.

- Use fabric softener on facecloths for gentle cleansing care.

- Moisturize under-eye skin more often.

- Use moisturizer during airplane travel to counteract in-flight dryness.

- Use a sunscreen product before prolonged sun exposure.

- Try to get 7 hours of sleep every night.

- Devote one evening a week to a total beauty ritual — facial sauna and facial masque, hair conditioning, manicure and pedicure.

1

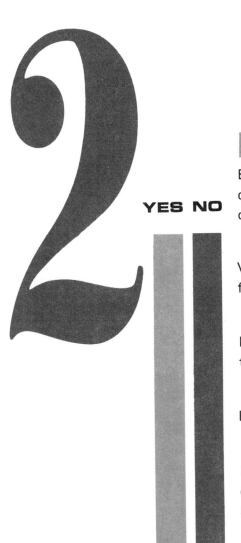

TREAT YOUR SKIN TO SOLUBLE COLLAGEN

YES NO

Below are some questions that will help you determine if your skin needs the special benefits of soluble collagen:

Would you like to refine or improve the look and feel of your skin?

Does your skin sometimes look and feel tight, taut or parched?

Does your skin lack vibrance and luster?

Do you have dry lines or wrinkles around your eyes, mouth or forehead due to premature aging?

Does the surface of your skin feel harsh, rough or uneven to the touch?

Do you experience dry flaking on your skin?

Is your skin beginning to lose its firmness?

If you answered "yes" to three or more of these questions, your skin could use the proven benefits of a soluble collagen-enriched beauty treatment. **Soluble collagen is the protein ingredient vital to firm, young skin.** It will improve the look of the skin and refine the skin surface so it feels significantly smoother. What's more, it effectively minimizes the appearance of premature dry lines and wrinkles.

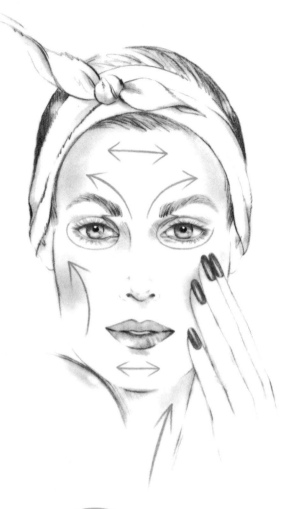

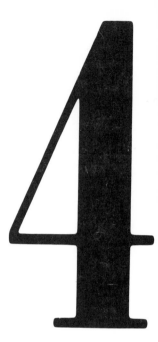

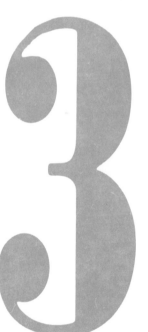

APPLY A FACE-LIFTING TOUCH

The way you apply skin care creams or lotions can help keep your face fit and firm. Beauty products should be smoothed on with finger-tips in an upward, outward direction as shown in the illustration. Using this method of touch helps counteract the natural force of gravity which pulls your face on a downward sag. When it comes to visible lines on the forehead, remember to go with the flow. Apply creams in the direction that lines are formed and massage outward toward the temples.

Use your ring finger to pat on eye creams, since it provides the softest touch. Be sure to moisturize your neck properly too. That is, start at your collarbone and work up and out to the jawline.

FADE AWAY PROBLEMS WITH FADE CREAM

Sun exposure emphasizes freckles and skin discolorations, since the color contrast between the spots and unaffected areas increases. When these darkened spots become more noticeable, a fade cream can visibly help. The most effective fade creams contain an ingredient called hydroquinone as well as sunscreen. Fade creams gradually lighten "liver spots" in some individuals, as well as skin discolorations caused by birth control pills and pregnancy. But whatever your needs, consistent use over a period of at least 6 weeks is vital to achieve the results you want.

66 The future of your face looks better than ever. Research and technology will bring about even more effective beauty creams. Each day chemists work to develop new sources of help for skin — "super creams" that retexturize the skin's surface, add elasticity and vibrancy, and help accelerate cell renewal. **99**

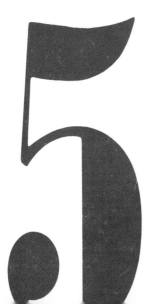

FOCUS ON EYE TREATMENT

The area around your eyes is very delicate, so fine lines and wrinkles are apt to show up there before they do on other areas of your face. Special care is necessary to help prevent these lines from forming as well as minimize the appearance of those that already exist. There are eye treatment products in both oil, lotion and cream forms.* Choose a lightweight texture to wear during the day under your makeup and a richer one to moisturize during the night.

*ALWAYS pat on your eye treatment with your ring finger. Begin at the outer corner of your eye and work inward toward your nose.

29

Before you do anything, create a relaxing atmosphere for yourself — the idea being to give yourself a beauty treatment inside and out. Spray the room with a floral fragrance. Turn on your favorite music, and proceed with Step 1. **Be sure to use these two steps in correct sequence.**

INTENSIFIED CLEANSING CARE

1.sauna

Face steaming is a pleasant and effective method of deep-cleaning your skin. The steam expands the pores and helps to draw out hard-to-reach impurities. How often you need to steam-bathe your face depends on you and your skin type. Oily skin, however, requires more frequent steam baths than drier skin. Before you start, cleanse your face thoroughly. Then follow these steps for a refreshing facial cocktail.

- Pour boiling water into a medium-sized bowl or your bathroom basin.

- Lean over water, close enough to feel the steam. Place a towel over your head to tent-in vapors and direct steam to your face for 3 to 5 minutes.

When facial sauna is not followed by a masque, rinse your face with cool water. Then apply toner and moisturizer.

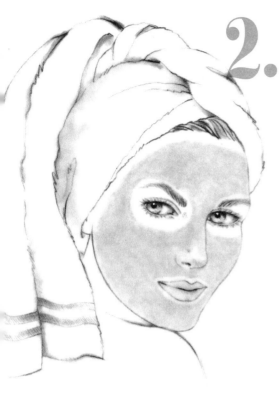

2. masque

The major function of a masque is to deep-clean, stimulate blood circulation and remove dead skin cells. Specifically, there are masques that cleanse, refine, retexturize, firm and moisturize. No one masque is right for you all the time. Climate, changes in your skin and lifestyle dictate the kinds of masques you need. But generally, these guidelines apply:

DRY AND MATURE SKIN — moisturizing masque

NORMAL/COMBINATION SKIN — various masques, according to your skin's particular characteristics and needs

OILY SKIN — deep-cleansing and/or refining/ retexturizing masque — depending on the current condition of your skin

To apply masque, read product directions. After thoroughly removing your makeup, smooth masque across forehead, nose and chin. Avoid eye and lip areas. Apply in upward strokes on the cheeks.

> 66 To help avoid the eye area, smooth eye cream around your eyes before applying the masque. 99

Now, stretch out on your bed with feet up to reverse circulation. Free your mind and concentrate on happy, pleasant thoughts. After the specified time, remove masque according to product directions. Then, follow with your after-cleansing toner and moisturizer. Your skin should look and feel soft, clean and radiant.

SENSITIVE OR ALLERGIC SKIN

If you develop one mystifying disorder after another:

- ■ Consult a dermatologist.
- ■ Cleanse gently to avoid irritating your skin.
- ■ Always use mild, fragrance-free products.
- ■ Use lightweight, water-rinsable products.

SOLUTIONS FOR PROBLEM SKIN

ACNE-PRONE SKIN

IF you're plagued by habitual skin eruptions,

BECAUSE hormonal disturbance or excessive oil production causes blockage and eventually inflammation in the pores and glands,

THEN take this expert advice:

- ■ Cleanse your face scrupulously at least 3 times a day with a gentle cleansing product.

- ■ Use a clean washcloth or face brush to dislodge oil from pores.

- ■ Use a full-strength toner with alcohol.

- ■ Use a medicated skin care product that contains benzoyl peroxide.

■ Use a light, oil-blotting moisturizer and face makeup for added protection during the day.

■ Apply a clay masque once or twice a week for intensified cleansing.

■ Consult a dermatologist to manage serious problems with breakout.

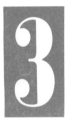

ADULT ACNE

When you're well beyond adolescence, and looking and feeling your best, a surprise attack of acne is understandably upsetting. Why is your skin acting up now?

Adult acne can arise for a number of reasons:

● A change in hormonal activity

● Medications taken internally

● A stressful job or situation

Sometimes acne develops after discontinuing estrogen-supplemented birth control pills. Estrogen helps arrest acne and when this added dose is eliminated from the body, hormonal changes occur that can bring on blemishes. Many acne disorders can be controlled with nonprescription treatments. Read labels and choose products that contain either precipitated sulfur, salicylic acid or benzoyl peroxide. Benzoyl peroxide seems to work best. If your acne doesn't respond to your time and efforts, consult a dermatologist for professional advice.

Adult acne is sometimes referred to as "chin acne" since breakout usually flares up around the chin.

SKIN CARE GLOŚ·SA·RY

acne
A disorder of the skin caused by inflammation of the skin's oil glands and hair follicles.

antiseptic
An antibacterial substance that inhibits the growth or action of germs and helps control infections.

benzoyl peroxide
An ingredient found in many acne-related products that helps to correct breakouts.

blackhead
An accumulation of blocked oil and skin pigment in an oil gland that is open to the surface of the skin.

collagen
A protein ingredient found in the connective tissue within the dermis that gives skin its youthful resiliency, firmness and moisture-retention capabilities.

dermis
The second layer of skin which contains blood vessels, oil and sweat glands, hair follicles, connective tissues, collagen and elastin fibers.

emollient
A skin-softening ingredient that adds to and helps retain moisture in the skin.

epidermis — The surface layer of skin where new cells are constantly being formed and where the living cells that produce melanin are contained.

humectant — An ingredient, usually in a moisturizer, that attracts and absorbs moisture from the air.

hydroquinone — An ingredient usually found in fade or bleaching creams that helps to lighten dark spots.

melanin — A dark brown or black pigment in skin and hair.

salicylic acid — An ingredient found in some products that helps fight blackheads and whiteheads.

sebaceous gland — The glands on the skin that secrete sebum (oil).

sebum — An oil secreted by the skin.

SPF — A term meaning Sun Protection Factor, which is found on many sunscreen products and is usually followed by a number which denotes the amount of time you can safely bathe in the sun.

toner — An after-cleansing product, also referred to as a freshener or astringent, that removes excess oils and cleanser residue and promotes a refined, youthful-looking skin texture.

T-zone — A term used to describe the forehead, nose and chin area, where oil glands tend to be the most productive.

ultraviolet — The invisible light rays that penetrate the epidermis and have been known to cause premature aging and skin cancer.

whitehead — An accumulation of oil in an oil gland that is trapped underneath the surface of the skin.

facecoloring,

like an applied art,

is based on artistic

principles:

PROPORTION

BALANCE

COMPOSITION

COLOR

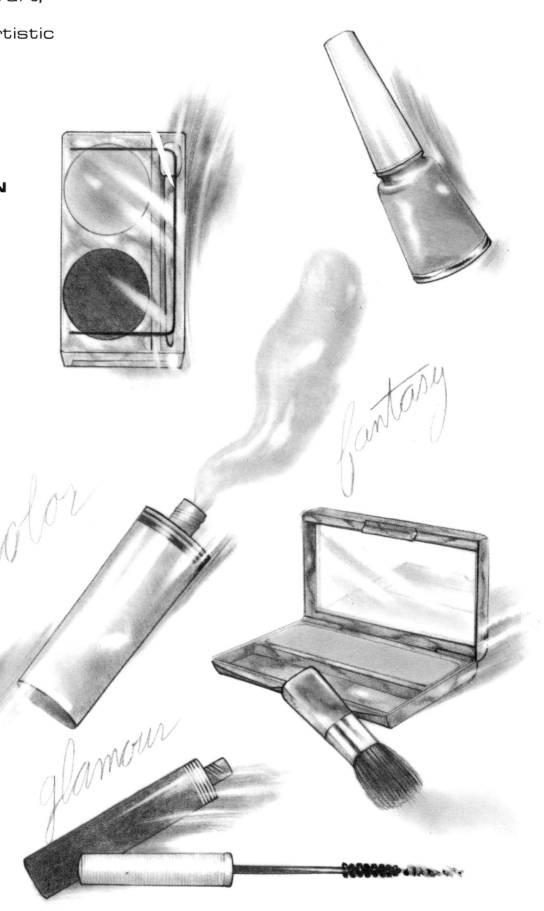

color

fantasy

glamour

MAKEUP 2.

FEATURE ATTRACTIONS IN FACECOLORING

MAKEUP is Magic. Creativity. Fun. And not as difficult a task as you may think. Makeup can be a love affair.

THINK of yourself as your own sculptor. It's you who must create and shape and mold yourself into the best that you can be. That's why educating yourself to your facial structure and your features is essential to discovering the makeup options and techniques that enhance you the most. Color, of course, is the creative key.

WHEN used cleverly, color creates illusion. Because color is emotion, glamour and fantasy. There are colors that lush the lips with outspoken sparkle. Shadows that bring to light the excitement of the eyes. Blushers that dramatize and accentuate the cheeks. The catchword is **experiment.** With practice, you'll develop the kind of quick-change talent and precision that will make you your own best beauty artist.

TEST

FACE-UP TO FACE-SHAPE

   1. Look into a mirror. Pull hair away from your face.

   2. Then compare the shape of your face to the illustrations and check the face shape that's most like yours.

FACE SHAPE = BEAUTY GEOMETRY

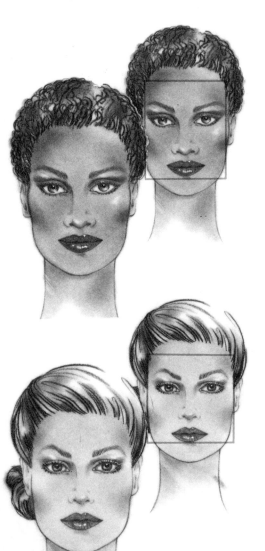

Your facial structure is a frame of reference — a base from which to take off. Face shape determines four primary beauty points which you will be reading about throughout this book:

1 The placement of makeup
2 Where and how to use contouring color
3 The hairstyles that look best on you
4 The shape of your eyeglasses

■ RECTANGULAR

The rectangular face is an elongated square shape. Forehead is about the same width as cheekbones and jawline.

■ SQUARE

The square face has a squared forehead about the same width as cheekbones and jawline. The squared jaw is the dominant feature.

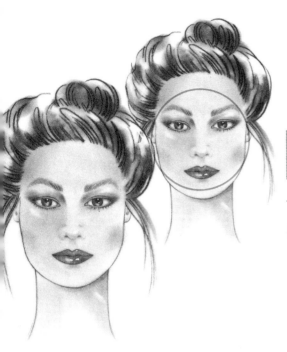

ROUND

The round face is almost as wide as it is long, with the greatest width at the cheeks.

TRIANGULAR

A triangular face has a wide forehead and high cheekbones. The triangular face tapers to a narrow chin.

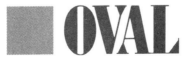# OVAL

The ideal face. Forehead is wider than the chin, cheekbones are dominant and the face gracefully tapers from cheeks to a narrower oval chin.

WHAT IT DOES FOR YOU. Foundation makes you look better. It evens out skin tone, veils imperfections and can actually do your skin a service: **1.** Offers a fitting base for other makeup products. **2.** Helps shield your skin from air pollutants and reduces the effects of sun and wind. **3.** Helps blot oil and reduce moisture loss. The result is clearer, healthier-looking skin.

THE FACTS ABOUT FOUNDATION

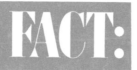

THERE ARE DIFFERENT FORMULAS. The kind of foundation you choose depends on the finished result you wish to achieve. Consider, too, your skin type and its visible condition.

FINISH
DEWY — Provides a moist, glowing finish
SEMI-MATTE — Natural-looking finish, neither moist nor powdery
MATTE — Velvety finish, free from shine

COVERAGE
SHEER — Transparent, see-through color that evens out skin tone but allows the beauty of skin to show through
MEDIUM — Coverage that masks minor imperfections and evens out skin tone while permitting some natural skin tone to show through
FULL — Conceals most flaws and imperfections

TYPE
LIQUID vs. CREAM — Both forms are available in all finishes and with varying degrees of coverage. Generally, cream formulas tend to produce a dewier finish and greater coverage. Cream foundations are usually more emollient and suggested for drier skins.

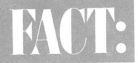

FOUNDATION SHOULD BE TAILORED TO YOUR SKIN TYPE FOR BETTER PERFORMANCE

FOR DRY SKIN Use a foundation fortified with moisturizers.

FOR SENSITIVE SKIN Use unfragranced makeup formulas.

FOR CLEAR SKIN Use a tinted moisturizer or a sheer foundation for transparent color and glow.

FOR OILY SKIN Use a water-based liquid makeup supplemented with oil-blotting ingredients to help refine the look and texture of your skin.

FOR BLEMISHED SKIN The options: Use a water-based full-coverage makeup or a medicated cover-up product applied to blemishes before your foundation.

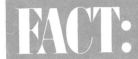

IT'S IMPORTANT TO FINE-TUNE FOUNDATION TO YOUR SKIN TONE. Before you buy a foundation, test it for color compatibility with your complexion. Foundation should be as close to your natural skin tone as possible. Apply it to your face, jawline or the inside of your wrist. Smooth on moisturizer first, since anything you use along with your makeup will affect its color.

Foundation is available in rose to peach to beige tones that range from light to medium to deep for darker skin. While foundation should match your complexion, slight variations may be necessary. For example, if your skin tends toward the sallow side, choose a slightly rosy foundation and blusher to counteract the yellow cast. For a ruddy skin tone, use beige or brown tones to play down the red. Avoid rose, red and pink blusher—peach, amber and brown are more flattering to ruddy coloring.

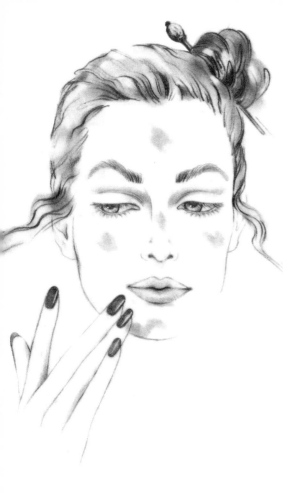

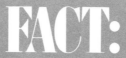

FACT:

BLEND FOUNDATION FOR THE BEST EFFECT. The cardinal rule: There should never be a noticeable line between you and your makeup. Blending is the answer to a natural-looking foundation finish. While application varies slightly from one makeup type to another, some pointers always hold true.

NORMAL TO DRY TO VERY DRY SKIN: Always use a moisture makeup.

OILY SKIN: Always use a water-based makeup and blend quickly before it dries.

APPLICATION TECHNIQUES

NORMAL TO VERY DRY SKIN:
- Start with a small amount dotted on forehead, nose, cheeks and chin.
- Blend well with long, light strokes in an outward direction extending to outer corners of your face and over jawline.

OILY SKIN:
- Start with a small amount dotted on forehead only and quickly blend.
- Then use the same procedure — one part of the face at a time — on nose, cheeks and chin.
- Blend immediately with long, light strokes in an outward direction to outer corners of your face and over jawline.

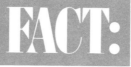

FACT:

CORRECT WITH CONCEALER: Eye concealers, whether in stick, cream, vial or pot form, neatly cover dark areas under the eyes as well as blemishes on the face. For best results, select the shade lighter than your natural skin tone. Be certain to apply after moisturizing and before foundation.

PERFECT WITH FACE POWDER

Loose powder or pressed powder can be worn with or without a makeup base. Like any foundation product, always select powder in the shade closest to your natural skin tone. Pressed powder is portable so use it throughout the day to pat away shine.

HOW DOES FACE POWDER ENHANCE YOUR FACE LOOKS? Helps makeup wear longer ● Blots away excess oil ● Freshens your appearance ● Creates a clear matte finish

---

Shake powder puff after each use to prevent powder glaze and oil buildup.

IS YOUR POWDER A PRO? After 4 to 6 hours' wear, evaluate the physical condition of the powder on your face.

● Does your face look shiny?

● Has powder streaked or caked?

● Has powder changed color?

THE BEST WAY TO BLUSH

Face shape determines the proper placement of blusher. Illustrated here are fundamental directions in cheek coloring based on bone structure. Learn the basic techniques before graduating to more sophisticated looks.

Generally, smaller faces look best with more vivid blusher colors, while subtle tones help slim down a full face.

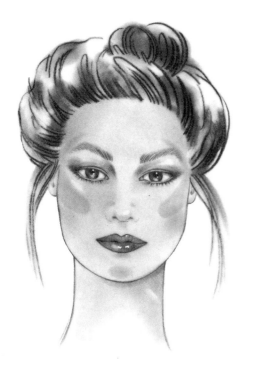

ROUND

Apply blusher in a sideways V on cheekbone, as shown, for a slenderizing effect. Blend up from cheekbone to temples. Then apply a touch of blusher to your chin and blend to give your face an added illusion of length.

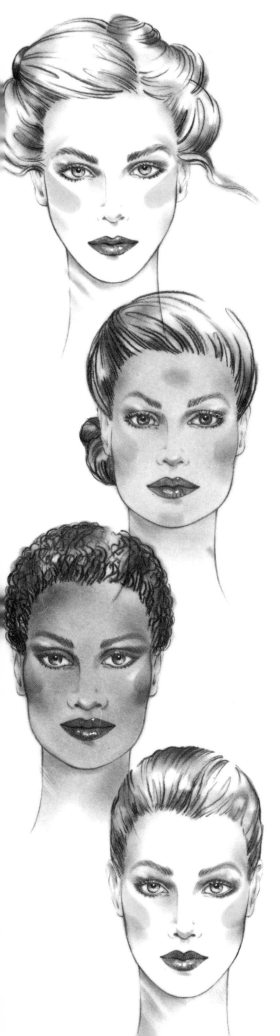

TRIANGULAR

Apply blusher in a sideways V on cheekbone. Blend up from cheekbone to temples, then extend over the eyebrow a bit toward the center of the forehead. This technique will help to balance the width of your forehead with the rest of your face. Avoid applying blusher on your chin.

SQUARE

Apply blusher on cheekbone, beginning at the center of the eye. Blend toward temple and apply a dab to forehead and chin to soften the square angle of your face.

RECTANGULAR

Apply blusher on cheekbone below outer corner of eye and blend up to temple to give more width to your face. Be sure blusher never extends lower than the tip of your nose.

OVAL

Find the most prominent part of your cheekbone, using your fingertips. Apply blusher at that point and blend up toward temples to highlight your cheekbone.

Blushers bring out the character in your face by giving bone structure more definition. The type of blusher you should use depends on your skin type and the finished look you want to achieve. But whatever blusher you select, one rule remains the same: Color-key your blusher to your lipstick for a harmonizing effect.

BASICS ABOUT BLUSHERS

What's the difference between cream and powder blushers?

cream blusher

1 Smooths on with your fingertips.
2 Gives skin a moist, dewy finish.
3 Looks and wears well on dry or normal-to-dry skin types.
4 Should be applied over foundation and before face powder.

powder blusher

1 May be applied with a brush, sponge or puff.
2 Looks and behaves well on all skin types, particularly oily skin.
3 Should be applied over foundation before or after face powder.

CHEEK SCULPTURING

Contouring is a basic principle of light and shadow — light projects and shadow recedes. Skillful contouring brings attention to your cheekbones and gives your face a more sculp-

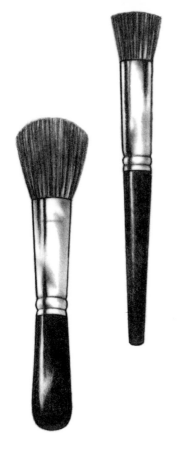

tured look. If you are not blessed with high cheekbones, you can create the illusion that you are. Creating more sophisticated cheek coloring looks does not mean using a heavy hand. As a matter of fact, since more elements are used, delicacy is essential. Discover new ways of working color, textures and design to bring special interest to your cheeks. <u>Think artistically</u> and couple colors that harmonize, not only with themselves but with lipcolor as well. Avoid colors that are too great a contrast for your natural skin tone. But whatever color or colors you use, blend well to create a natural finish.

CONTOUR WITH COLOR

Using two tones of the same color — one light, one darker — apply deeper shade under your cheekbone in the hollow area and the lighter shade above it so that they're side by side. Then lightly blend to an even-toned look. This technique creates the illusion of more prominent cheekbones.

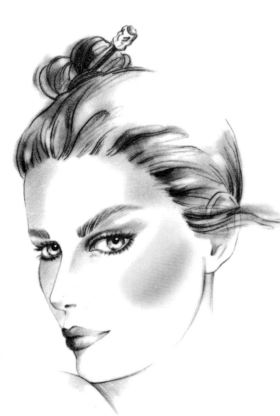

CONTOUR WITH TEXTURE

Pair a darker matte blusher with a lighter frosted blusher. Apply darker matte color in the hollow area under your cheekbone. Then sweep the lighter frosted blusher above it so that they're side by side. This technique makes cheekbones appear higher. Blend carefully — you should never see where one blusher shade begins and the other ends.

TEST

1 Color your lips within their exact lip line.

2 Blot lips with a tissue, being careful to pick up exact lip outline.

3 Compare tissue tracing to lip shapes in the following chart and check the one that's most like yours.

4 Or, simply kiss this page for an on-the-spot evaluation.

SHAPING-UP YOUR LIPS

When it comes to makeup, lipstick is on the most-wanted list. If you're like the majority of women, it's the most frequently used item in your bag of beauty tricks. And the one that you feel the most comfortable using. But there's a lot more to lips than lipstick.

Now follow the directions for your lip shape to make your mouth more symmetrical.

NORMAL LIPS

Since your lips are naturally symmetrical, corrective measures don't apply to you. Experiment as you please with lipcolors and textures to create different effects.

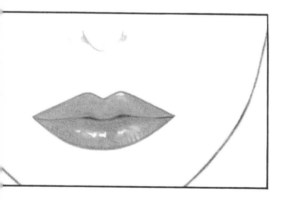

FULL LIPS

Apply a small amount of face makeup over mouth. Use lip liner just inside natural lip line, defining corners as well. Use soft, medium-to-dark cream lipcolor. Apply carefully to outer corners of mouth. Avoid bright colors, frosts and glosses.

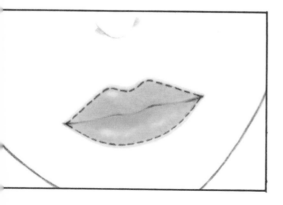

THIN LIPS

Use lip liner to outline your mouth along the outer edge of the natural lip line. Give a fuller look by using light-to-medium colors, frosts and glosses.

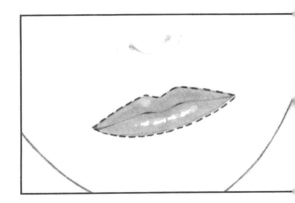

FULLER TOP LIP
FULLER BOTTOM LIP

There are two options:
You can make your fuller lip look thinner or your thinner lip appear fuller. Use lip liner on both lips.

TO EMPHASIZE thinner lip, apply lip liner along <u>outer</u> edge of your natural lip line. Then fill in both lips with a bright shade of lipcolor.

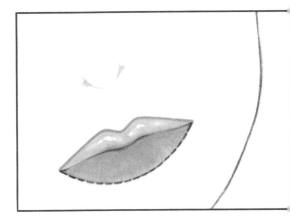

TO DE-EMPHASIZE fuller lip, apply lip liner along the <u>inner</u> edge of your natural lip line. Then fill in both lips with a dark lipcolor.

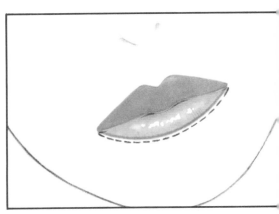

DROOPING LIPS

Cover the corners of your mouth with face makeup or concealer. Use lip pencil to subtly extend lip corners upward. Then fill in color.

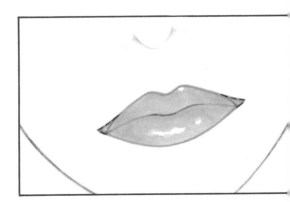

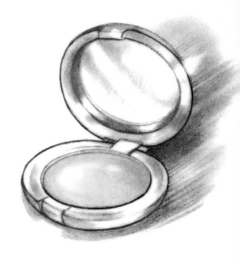

PRONOUNCED EFFECTS FOR LIPS

Lip makeup comes in more forms and colors than one can talk about. The difference is the kind of coverage and shine they offer. Once you understand these various effects, you'll be able to make the expert choices that do the most for you. Lipcolor tip: light color and gloss emphasize. Dark color and matte finish de-emphasize.

PRODUCT CATEGORIES

FROSTS
Colors that contain shimmering qualities and create a soft glazed effect

CREAMS
Colors with no noticeable pearl or frosted qualities that give the lips a creamy, moist look

GLOSSES
Colors lushed with high-gloss shine, usually sheer in coverage

SHEERS OR TRANSPARENTS
Clear or tinted coverage, with glossy shine that lets your own natural lipcolor show through

PRODUCT FORMS

SWIVEL TUBES
The classic form of lipcolor, swivel tubes are the most popular lipstick applicator

PENCILS
Three types — those that line lips, those that fill in color, and dual-purpose that do both

VIALS
Abundant combination of color and shine usually applied with a sponge-tip applicator

POTS OR COMPACTS
Sheer, shiny lipcolor applied with fingertips

LIFEGUARDS FOR LIPS Keeping lips soft, smooth and moist-looking requires a bit of **TLC** — Tender Lip Care. Treat your lips to a specially formulated lip moisturizer. Wear it at bedtime or under lipcolor. Use sunscreen in the sun and products that protect lips from the drying touch of cold and wind.

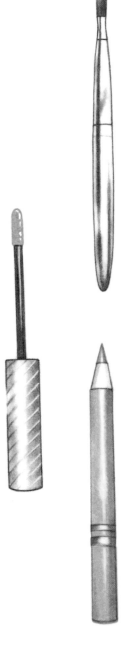

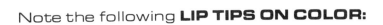

Note the following **LIP TIPS ON COLOR:**

- For longer-wearing lipstick, apply foundation and/or face powder on lips before using lip liner and color.

- Use a lip pencil in the same shade as your lipstick or slightly deeper.

- Use a lip brush for more precise application and to vary depth of color.

- For dark skin: If natural lipcolor is uneven, use a lip lightener or darkener before applying color.

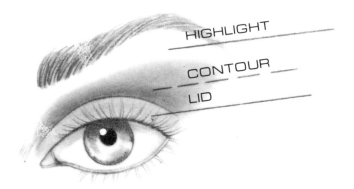

HIGHLIGHT

CONTOUR

LID

FOCUS ON YOUR NAKED EYE

More than any other feature, eyes are in plain sight and give your face energy, excitement and individuality. Skillful application of color is essential, since eye makeup mistakes have a pronounced effect on your overall appearance. Get to know what shape your eyes are in and the basic technique you should follow before you attempt any elaborate shadowing. Look into a mirror and compare your eyes to the illustrations here. Choose the eyes that most resemble yours. Then follow the how-to advice. Refer to it for basic direction when designing your own private eye ideas.

SMALL EYES

- For an eye-opener, apply frosted or pastel color on eyelid
- Use a darker color in the contour crease
- Highlight area under the brow with a frosted shade to give the eye more prominence

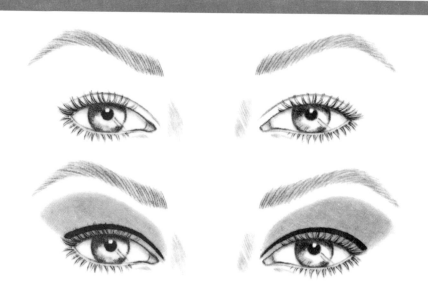

ALMOND EYES

- No makeup corrective is necessary so have fun experimenting
- Try a favorite shade on the lid and extend to contour area
- Apply a deeper tone of the same color to the outer corner of lid slanting outward just beyond the eye
- Blend a light shade under brow for highlighting

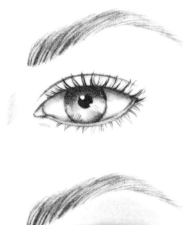
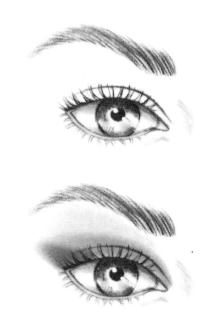
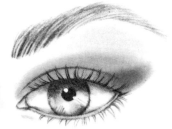

ORIENTAL EYES

- Apply a highlighter under the brow area
- Divide the remaining eye area in half vertically
- Use light, bright shadow color in the half closest to your nose
- And a darker, more subdued tone in the outer half

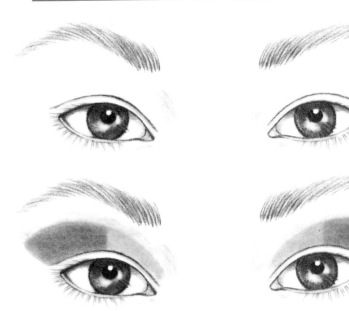

PROMINENT EYES

- To help recess the look of your eyes, apply a dark flat color to eyelid and extend into eye crease
- Use a flat pastel color under the brow for highlight

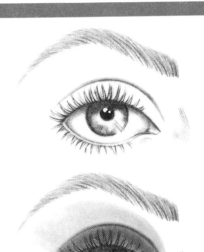
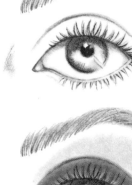
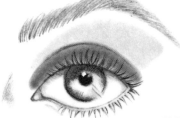

ROUND EYES

- To compliment the roundness of your eyes, apply two colors in a half circle — the lighter shade under your brow and a deeper tone beneath
- Or, elongate a round eye by wrapping it with color. Apply subtle, matte shade on lid and into contour crease. Extend the same matte shade to the outer eye corner and continue down along lower lid to just under the center of your eye

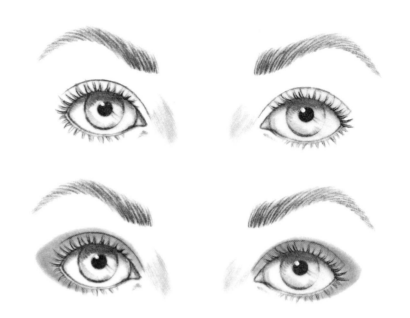

DEEP-SET EYES

- Try a halo effect to bring eyes out
- Use light, bright frosted colors on the eyelid and as highlighter under brow
- Use medium-to-dark color in the eye crease

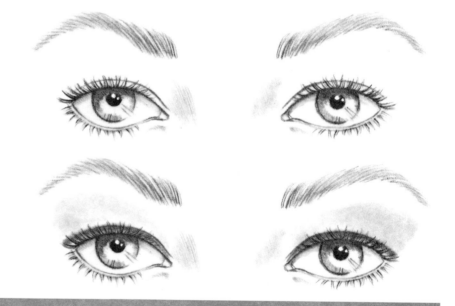

HOODED EYES

- Apply bright, frosted color on eyelid and extend to contour area
- Use a frosted or pastel highlighter directly under brow

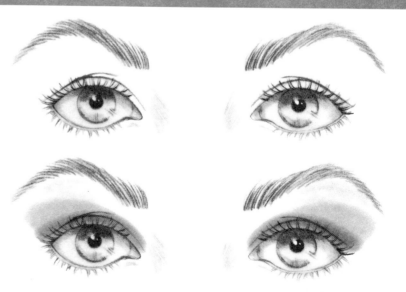

Fashion trends affect how you line or don't line your eyes. But whatever the current eye fashion, eyeliner does four basic things for your eyes:

1 Gives sharper definition to eye shape
2 Makes lashes look longer
3 Makes eyes look larger
4 Amplifies the whites of the eyes.

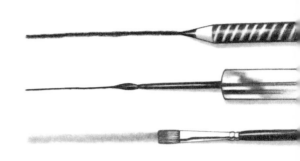

DRAMATIZING WITH EYELINER

Eyeliners come in various colors and forms: vial types, liquids, solid cakes and pencils.

Pencil eyeliners are versatile designers and can be used to create various effects:

● thinly applied for a fine, natural-looking line

● applied more intensely for a more dramatic impression

● blended or smudged for a soft, smoky look

Pencils are offered in every color you could ever wish to use. What's more, most women find pencils easier to control than a liquid or cake eyeliner product.

66 When applying eyeliner, remember to keep the line at the base of your lashes. Rest the heel of your hand against your chin for more skillful application. **99**

PENCIL POINTS ON EYELINER

1 Use a freshly sharpened pencil for a fine line.
2 For a smudged effect, use a sponge-tip shadow applicator, an eyeshadow brush or a blunt-pointed eye pencil.
3 When pencil is softer than you'd like, refrigerate before using.
4 When pencil is harder than you'd like, soften it a bit by holding the tip between your fingers a moment or two.

Your lashes do more than meet the eye. Frankly, they serve a seductive purpose. Lashes emphasize the way you move and blink your eyes and the mood in your eyes. And using mascara heightens the effect and drama.

THE MAKING OF LAVISH LASHES

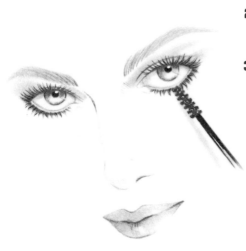

Basically, there are three types of mascara:

1 WATERPROOF: provides extra-long wear.

2 NATURAL LOOK: supplies subtle color that gives definition to lashes.

3 LASH BUILDERS: give length and thickness to lashes — often contain lash-like fibers.

To create more versatile eye looks, have three or four mascaras on hand — different types and different colors.

YOUR CHOICES

THE NEUTRALS:
BROWN ●BLACK ●CHARCOAL

THE FASHION SHADES:
PLUM ●VIOLET ●NAVY ●GREEN ●BURGUNDY

APPLICATION

When applying mascara, always hold wand in the way that's most comfortable for you to ensure better control. Brush on two to three coats, allowing drying time between each application. Use wand tip to coat bottom or shorter lashes at the corner.

PROBLEMS

- too pale
- too thin
- too short

- too sparse
- too straight
- too unruly

SOLUTIONS

1 If your lashes are short, sparse or thin (and lengthening/thickening mascara isn't enough), use false or individual lashes to add length and fullness. Remember to use natural-looking lashes for day, lavish types for night.

2 Use an eyelash curler to give straight lashes more shape and lift. Some lash curlers have a specially treated surface that allows you to use them before or after mascara is applied.

3 Use a lash comb or clean mascara brush to smooth out too thick or unruly lashes.

Reminders about mascara removers: Always use eye makeup remover to minimize pulling, wiping and rubbing delicate eye area. Waterproof mascara removes easily with a waterproof eye makeup remover.

LASH TIPS

▶ If you wear contact lenses, avoid mascara that contains lash-building fibers.

▶ Pep up pale lashes with vibrant color.

▶ Coordinate eyeliner and mascara colors for an interesting effect.

▶ Moisturize dry, brittle, delicate lashes with a lash conditioner at bedtime.

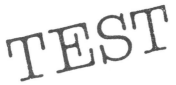

TEST

Brow shape is based on the placement
or spacing between your eyes.
To help you accurately determine
how your eyes are spaced, look into a mirror
and compare your eyes
to the illustrations.

HIGHBROW BEAUTY FOR EYES

Your eyebrows can alter the entire look of your face. When correctly shaped, they are as good as an expert makeover. If you find that your brows don't measure up, follow the instruction perfected for your eye spacing.

BROWS FOR CLOSE-SET EYES

- Start browline slightly in from the inner corner of eye
- Arch it just beyond the center of eye
- End slightly beyond the outer corner of eye

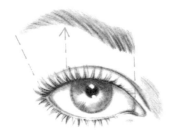

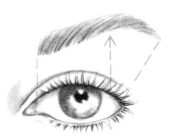

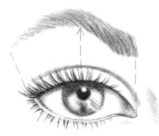

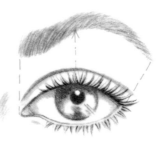

BROWS FOR WELL-SPACED EYES

- Start browline directly above inner corner of eye
- Arch it over center of eye
- End above outer corner of eye

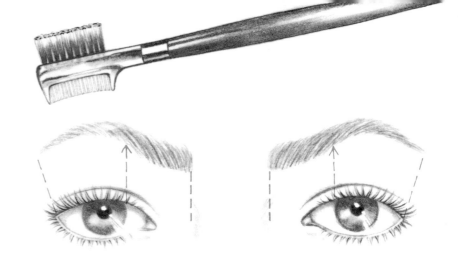

BROWS FOR WIDE-SPACED EYES

- Start browline slightly closer to nose than the inner corner of eye
- Arch slightly in front of the center of eye
- End above outer corner of eye

❝ If your brows are too light or too skimpy, feather on more color with a brow pencil. Then blend with brow brush to refine color and give a natural look.

For silky-looking brows, brush daily with a brow brush or soft toothbrush. **❞**

FOR BROWS THAT DON'T MEASURE UP

SKIMPY BROWS
- Use brow pencil in short feathering strokes to fill in brows.
- Then use a brow brush to blend in lines.

THICK BROWS
- To thin eyebrows, tweeze a few hairs across the length of brow.
- Be sure to pluck below browline, never above.

BUSHY OR UNRULY
- Brush brow down, then trim the tips with small round-ended scissors.
- Apply hairspray to brow brush before using to help tame brows.

BROW TIP:

When shaping brows, use an alternating technique. Tweeze a few hairs from one brow and then from the other. Using this back and forth pattern will help you achieve more perfectly balanced brows.

LIFE WITHOUT COLOR

DULL Imagine a world in shades of grey **DARK** the grey of the grass **BLAND** the grey of the sky **BLEAK** the grey of sunset **BARE** the grey of an orange **BLANK** nothing warm nothing cool **BR-R-R-R** relentless monotony **COLOR** so powerful in its presence, it can only be fathomed in its absence.

COLOR 3.

THE BEST SHADES OF YOUR LIFE

When light takes darkness by surprise, color unfolds and feelings flow. Because color is filled with energy and deep-felt presence. Revlon's impresarios create color to affect emotions, moods and attitudes.

CORAL is capricious. Some Revlon artists see coral as refreshingly impromptu. To them, it is as fickle and whimsical as a rainbow in a salmon sky.

PLUM is poignant. Revlon researchers feel that plum can be profound and poetic — a chromatic union of sensitivity and tenderness. Like the sigh of a seashell.

BLUE is bashful. True blue lovers at Revlon believe that the truest blue dwells in demure serenity: a butterfly poised on a petal, the tentative moment between day and dusk.

BROWN is brave. At Revlon, brown is a constellation of courage. It reflects the soaring strength of a journey on a winged horse. Handsome. Physical.

LILAC is lovesick. Many Revlon people imagine lilac as an emotion that wistfully languishes on the brink of love — a magical mood in which wishes are fulfilled.

RED is resolute. To Revlon colorists, red is exuberant. And dynamic. It is a color alive with rampant emotion and assured character. For these reasons, it became the Revlon signature color.

FIRST THERE WAS RED

THEN THERE WAS REVLON. Then there was dragon red, after dark red, shanghai scarlet, daring young red, tawny red, cherries in the snow, fifth avenue red, million dollar red, fire & ice, real red, red hot red, on-the-town red, raven red, gypsy fire, certainly red, cadillac red, love that red, bamboo red, softsilver red, saturday night red, years ahead red, sophisticated red, new wave red, mahogany red, brand new red.

AND THERE WAS PINK

AND THERE WAS REVLON. Then there was pink crystal, **pink spicing, shell pink, honeybee pink,** paint the town pink, **naked pink,** pink blush, **sphinx pink,** misty pink, **rose wine,** silvered rose, **seashell rose,** soft-silver pink, **rose indigo,** softshell pink, **desert pink frost,** love that pink, **ming rose,** butterfly pink, **passionata pink,** carioca pink, **pinkfoil,** silverpearl pink, **silver city pink,** coming up roses, **a rose is a rouge.**

MAGICAL, VIVID, LUSTROUS

COLOR creates magical effects. It has given bland skin natural-looking shine, purely natural color. Color has illuminated many a drab eye. Rubied lips to a kiss of perfection. And added a glowing cast from cheek to cheek.

The pages that follow are designed to make you your own impresario of color. The wide and vivid ranges of shades offer a never-ending spectrum of choices for the face.

To help you discover a diversity of makeup looks, upcoming pages feature the following elements:

● Six different face looks for everyone

● A range of fashion colors that complement each face look

● Five different eyeshadow techniques

● Practice pages for face and eyecolor experiments

BEFORE you try your hand at application techniques, you'll need an array of eyeshadows, lipcolors and 2 or 3 blushers for your makeup experiments.

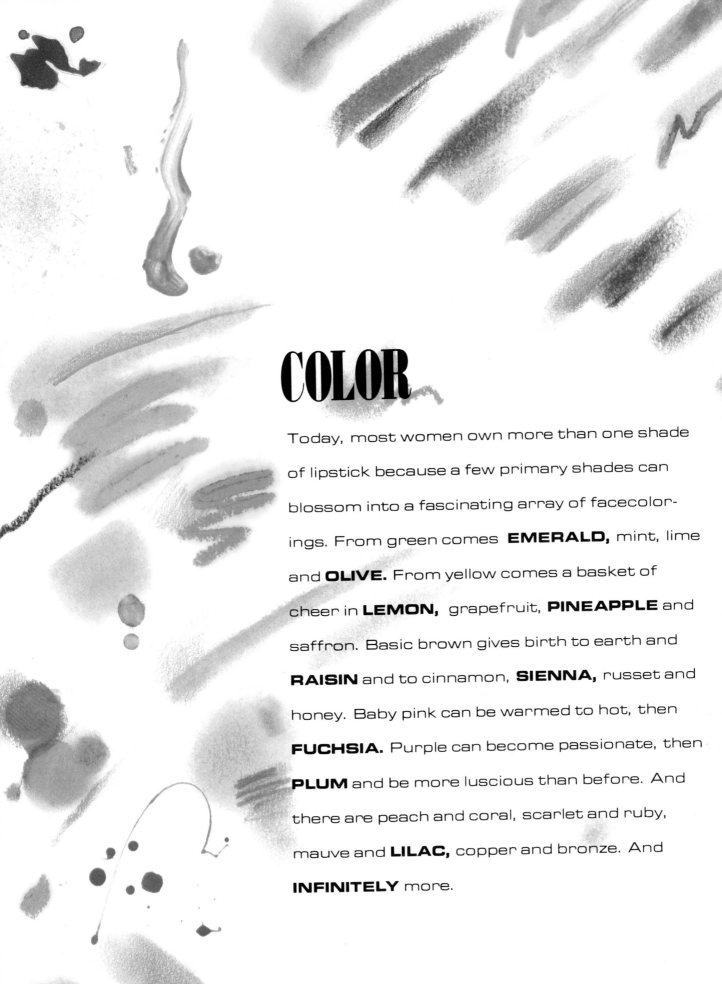

COLOR

Today, most women own more than one shade of lipstick because a few primary shades can blossom into a fascinating array of facecolorings. From green comes **EMERALD,** mint, lime and **OLIVE.** From yellow comes a basket of cheer in **LEMON,** grapefruit, **PINEAPPLE** and saffron. Basic brown gives birth to earth and **RAISIN** and to cinnamon, **SIENNA,** russet and honey. Baby pink can be warmed to hot, then **FUCHSIA.** Purple can become passionate, then **PLUM** and be more luscious than before. And there are peach and coral, scarlet and ruby, mauve and **LILAC,** copper and bronze. And **INFINITELY** more.

THE PINK/ROSE FACE

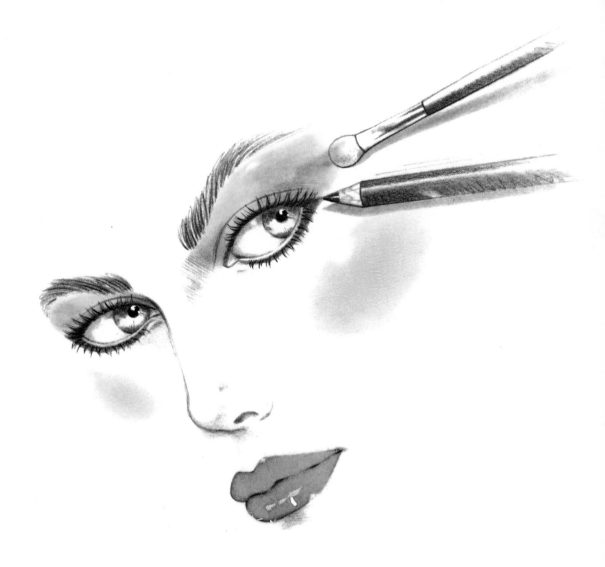

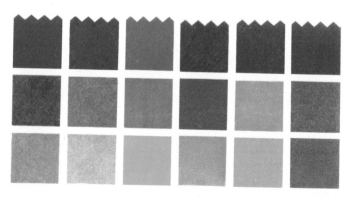

Coordinating Fashion Colors

THE PLUM/LILAC FACE

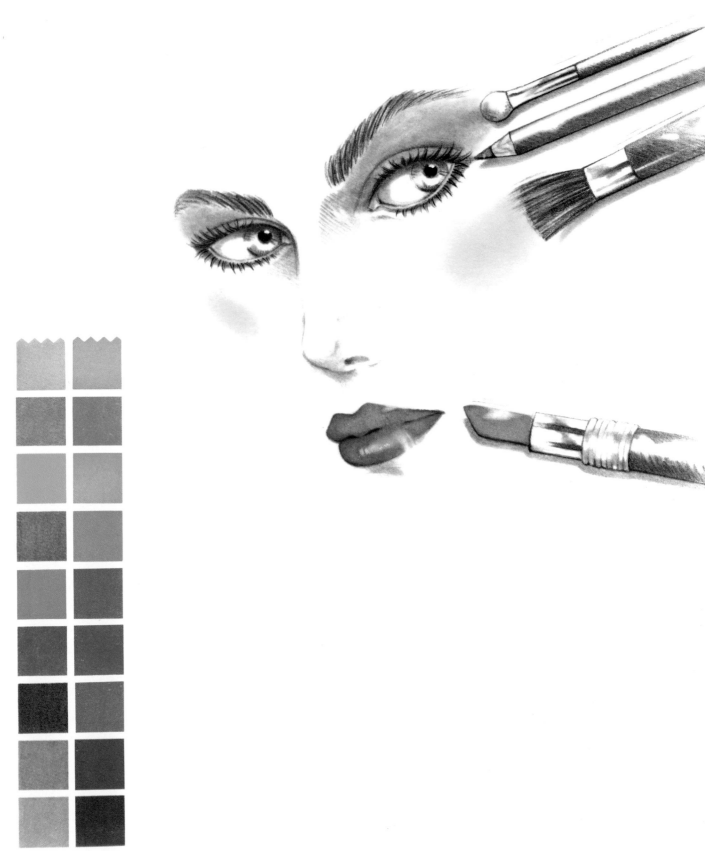

THE AMBER/BROWN FACE

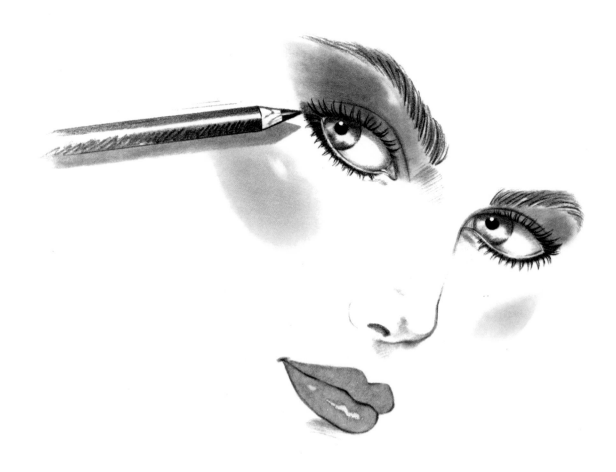

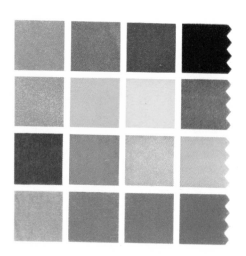

Coordinating Fashion Colors

THE CORAL/CINNAMON FACE

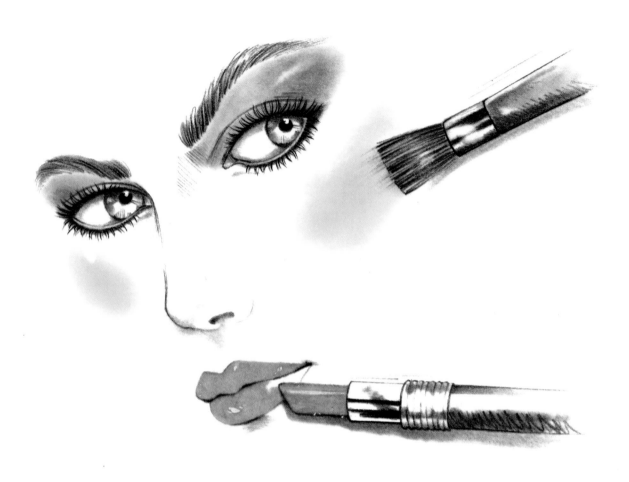

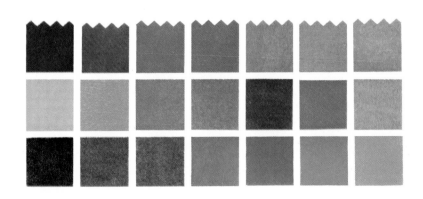

THE BLUE/BLUE FACE

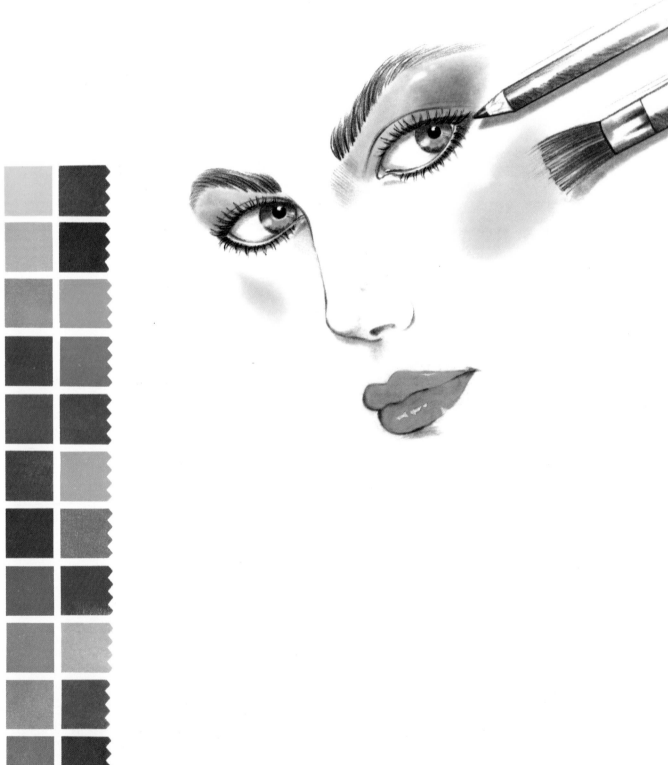

THE NEW NEUTRAL FACE

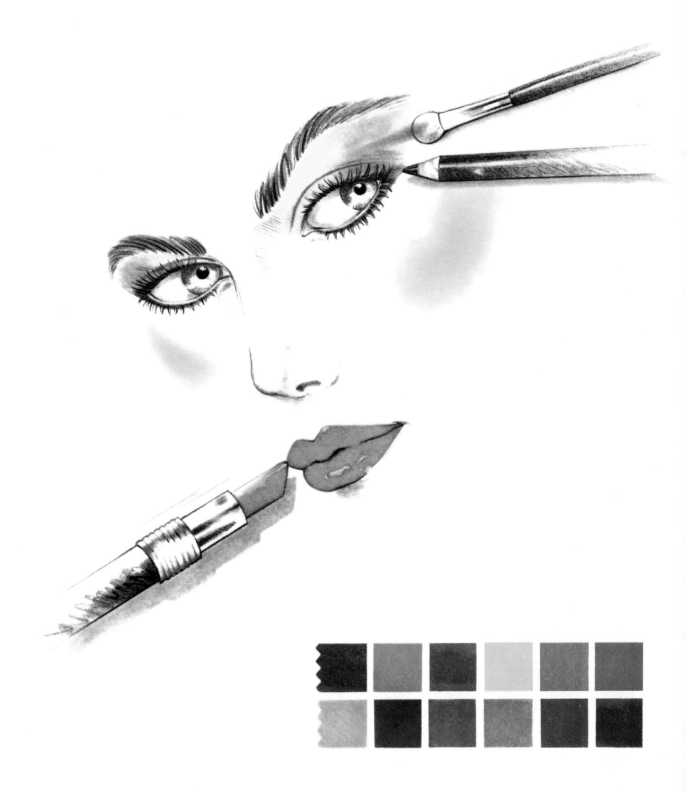

A WARDROBE OF EYE DESIGNS

THREE-TONED EFFECT

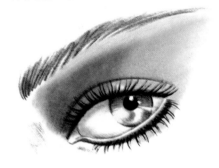

RAINBOW EFFECT

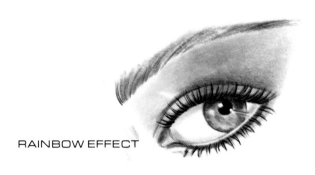

TWO-TONED EFFECT

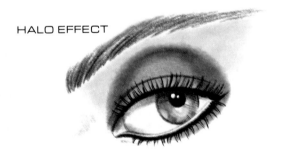

HALO EFFECT

HIGH CONTRAST EFFECT

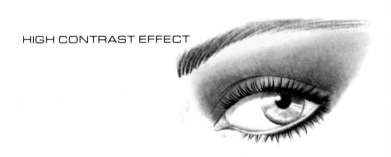

PARFAIT EFFECT

SPOTLIGHT EFFECT

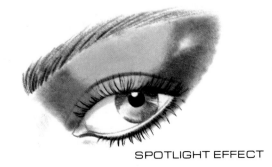

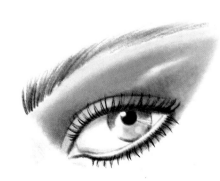

DESIGNS FOR DESIGNING EYES

To give your private eyes a little public spirit, **EXERCISE CREATIVITY** with eye makeup. The idea of matching shadow to your eyecolor is, happily, passé. Use color and technique to make your eyes more expressive, and to give them mood and magic. The palette of colors is as varied as a painter's paintbox.

When using 2 or 3 colors to create a **PARFAIT EFFECT,** be sure the colors are well blended and compatible. Then compose clever designs with pale and muted tones like taupe, olive, rose and mauve. Experiment with lush berry colors, plums, teals or jewels of jade, ruby and amethyst. Reserve brights like turquoise, fuchsia and starry violet for dramatic accent.

DARK SKIN TONES should avoid pastel eyecolors. The strong contrast between dark skin and pale colors can result in a contrived look.

66 EYESHADOW TIPS: Remove eyeshadow with products specified as eye makeup removers. Apply a special eyeshadow base to help eyecolors wear longer. **99**

Practice page eyecoloring

The eye drawings on these two pages are ready to color. Select at least four different eyeshadow shades to use as your palette. Try creating 2 or 3 of the EYE DESIGNS shown on page 72. Then practice coordinating colors into harmonious schemes. Two examples are indicated.

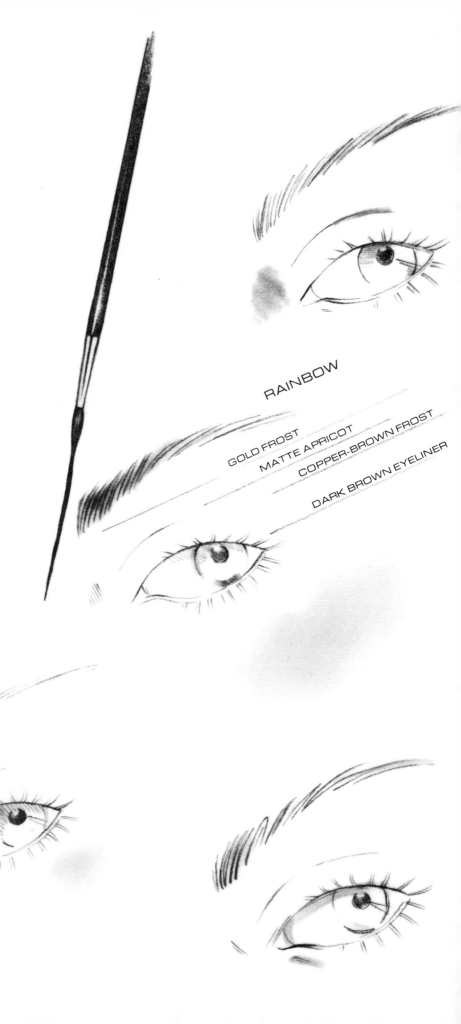

RAINBOW

GOLD FROST

MATTE APRICOT

COPPER-BROWN FROST

DARK BROWN EYELINER

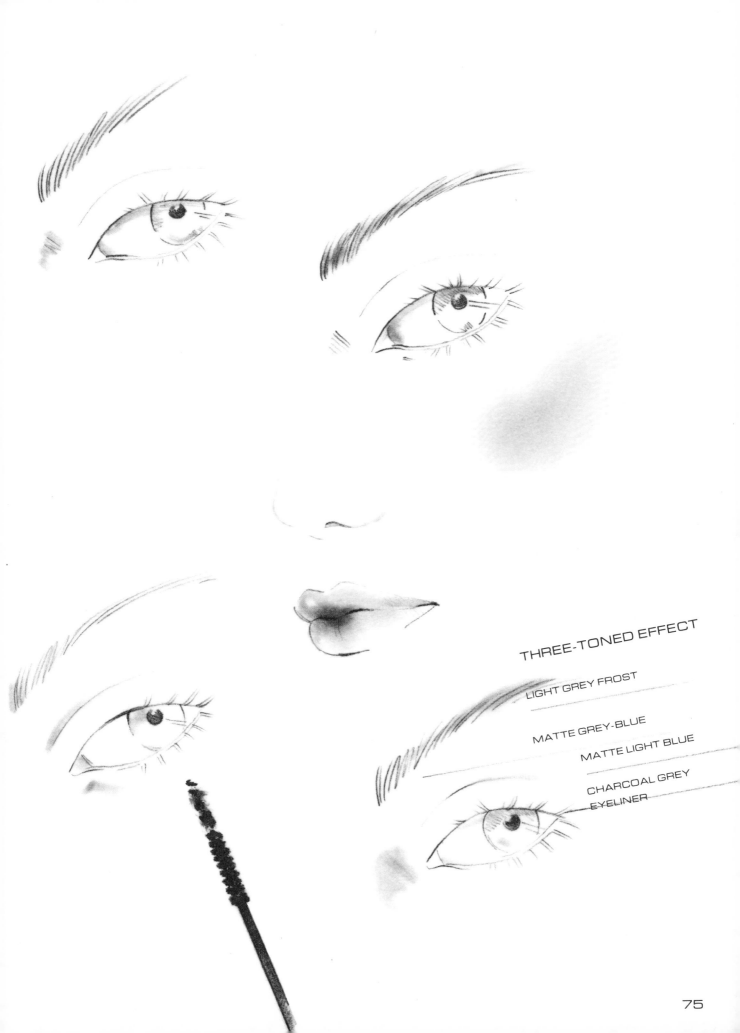

THREE-TONED EFFECT

LIGHT GREY FROST

MATTE GREY-BLUE

MATTE LIGHT BLUE

CHARCOAL GREY
EYELINER

Practice page facecoloring

The following faces are
ready to color. Makeup
to have on hand: a range
of eyeshadows, eyelining
pencils, blushers and
lipcolors. Try these
four palettes. Then
compose your own.

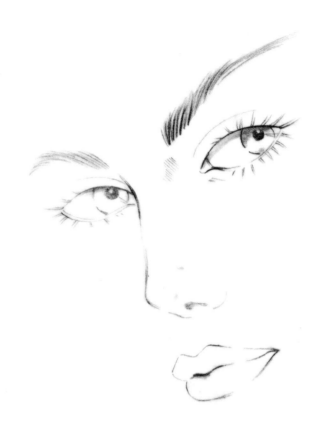

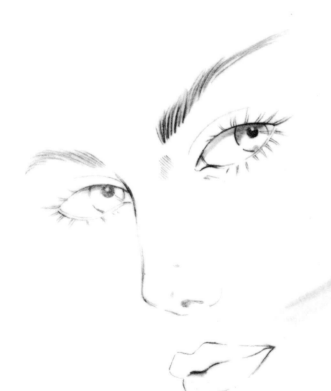

PALETTE 1

Pale pink highlighter under
brow • Grey-brown eye-
shadow • Dark brown or
black eyeliner • Soft red
blush • Red lipstick

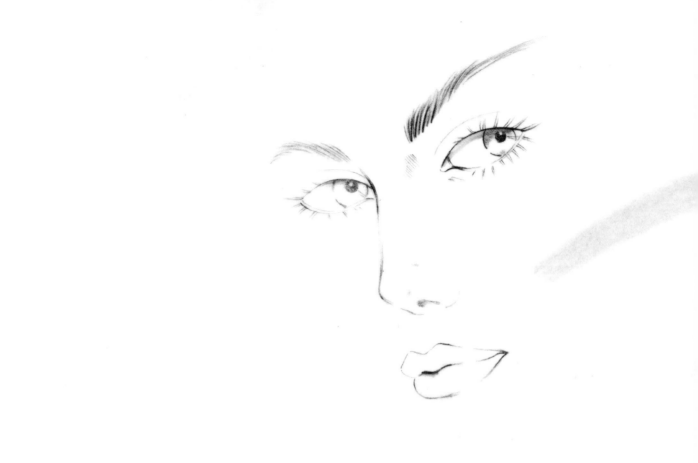

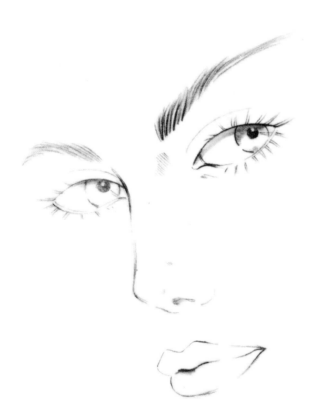

PALETTE 2

Pale peach highlighter
under brow • Russet eye-
shadow on inside half of eye
• Spruce green eyeshadow
on outside half of eye • Dark
green eyeliner • Russet
blush • Russet lipstick

PALETTE 3

Gold frost highlighter under
brow • Olive or forest green
eyeshadow • Dark green
eyeliner • Coral blush •
Sienna lipstick

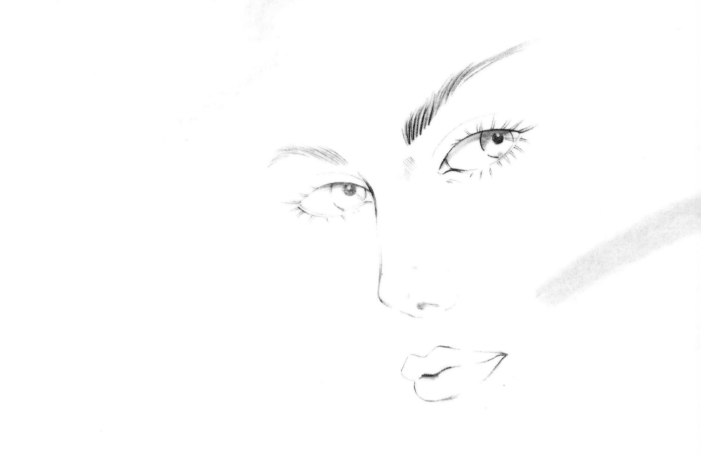

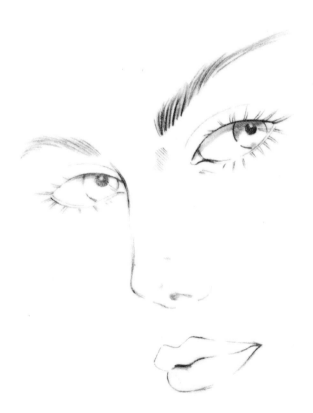

PALETTE 4

Pale lilac highlighter under brow • Vivid violet eyeshadow on inside half of eye • Dark plum eyeshadow on outside half of eye • Plum blush • Plum lipstick

UPDATE ON GLASS WEAR

Look around you. All kinds of people are looking spectacular with glasses. And why not? Glasses are a fashion accessory.

They come in great-looking colors and striking shapes to accentuate the face. And if you choose to, you can look at the world through **rose-colored glasses.** Or **yellow, blue or violet** for that matter. Here are some basic tips to help you make the choices that best complement your skin tone.

SELECTING YOUR COLOR

Pale, fair-skinned complexions are enhanced with warm colors. Select soft shades of **red, russet, sienna and tawny browns.**

Brown, olive or ruddy complexions should avoid colors that mimic natural skin tone. Paler frame shades, such as **blue and grey,** lend needed contrast to warm skin tones as will **brights.**

Complexions with a sallow yellow cast should avoid yellow frames and other shades with dominant yellow overtones, as the effect will intensify sallowness.

FRAMING YOUR FACE

When chosen correctly, glass wear can enhance face shape by improving its proportion and creating the illusion of balance.

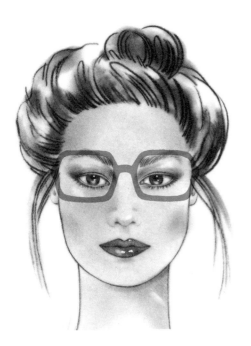

ROUND

Angular frames de-emphasize roundness. Choose styles that are slightly wider than the widest point of the face for a slimming effect. The bridge of the frames should be wide as well and somewhat arched.

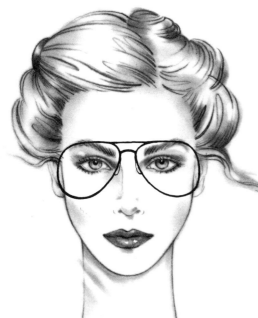

TRIANGULAR

To give better proportion to the face, keep the width of frames just within the temple hairline. The bridge should be softly curved and the lower half of the frame shaped in a downsweep.

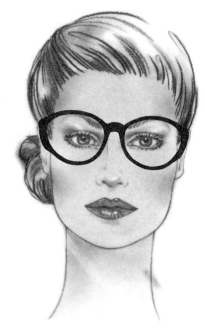

■SQUARE

Use gracefully curved frame shapes to relieve the angular structure of a square face. Frames should be slightly wider than the widest point of your jawline and the bridge arched. The lower part of the frame should sweep up toward the brow.

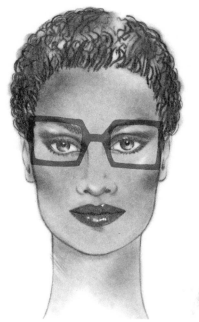

■RECTANGULAR

To create the illusion of a broader face, keep the overall width of frames within the border of the widest point of the cheekbones. The bridge of the frames should be slightly curved.

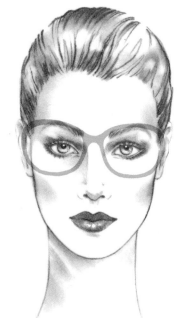

■OVAL

Because the oval face is an ideal shape, it's important not to detract from its natural beauty and symmetry. Experiment with varied frame looks to find the most suitable styles.

TIPS FOR BETTER FIT

How glasses fit the face is essentially determined by the bridge area of the frame. And the way this bridge is made can influence the look of certain facial features.

 To shorten a long nose, make sure the bridge of the frame is low.

 To slim a wide nose, choose glasses with a dark-colored bridge.

 To give width to close-set eyes, choose frames with a neutral-colored bridge.

 The tops of glasses should always cover eyebrows to eliminate the impression of two brows.

HINTS ON TINTS

Not all lens tints are recommended by opticians for regular or prolonged use in the sun. Pink may be your preferred color, but no matter how dark a pink or red tint, they offer little protection from ultraviolet rays. The same holds true for yellow and blue. Use grey, brown and green tints to filter out harmful rays.

QUICK TAKES ON BODY SHAPES

Like the face, your figure has a distinct structure and shape. And when body shape is not all it should be, alterations are necessary. As in makeup, the fashion theory is **light/bright colors project** and **dark/muted shades recede.** More women make mistakes picking the wrong shade than picking the wrong color. The shade of a color can make all the difference when it comes to flattering your figure. The following body shapes typify common figure problems.

CLOTHING COLOR AND CUT CAN PERFORM LIKE A BALANCING ACT ON THE BODY.

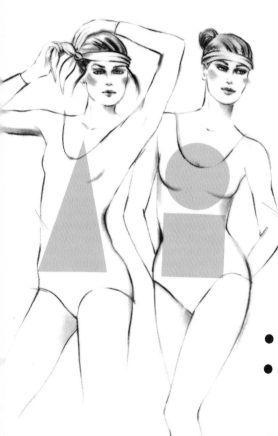

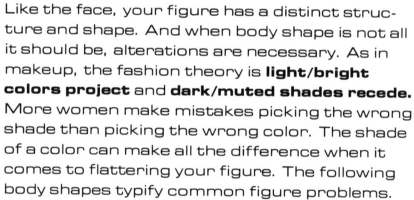

circle/square

The object here is to elongate and taper the rounder top portion of the body.

- Wear long, smooth-flowing tops.

- Stick to shades from the same color family for tops and bottoms to lengthen your overall appearance.

- Try a dark top under a light jacket to visibly deflate the circle shape.

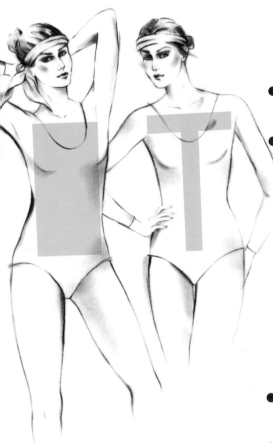

the triangle

The bottom-heavy figure has a gamut of optical illusions from which to choose.

● Yes, you can wear light-colored trousers. Just top them with a bright, blousy shirt, the idea being: What you wear on top should be more eye-catching than what you wear on the bottom part of your body.

● Pair pale bottoms with a lighter shade top or a pure white top.

● Stronger contrasting only works well if you remember to elongate the top portion of your body. Beware of chopping yourself in half with a top that falls short of the hips.

the rectangle

This straight up-and-down shape needs curving, and a particular kind of waist definition.

● Keep clothing shades monotone and redefine the waist with a brightly contrasting belt.

● Wear dark-colored pullover tops and accent with a slim belt in the same color to create a natural-looking curve.

the model T

Although long and linear, the T-shaped body can look meager in the wrong shade of a color.

● Wear light-colored outfits with a touch of bright accents to give your figure a boost.

● Soften your angular lines with blousy tops and dresses in light or bright colors.

hand exam

Can you positively answer "yes" to these questions?

1 Are your nails uniformly shaped and proportionate lengths?

2 Are your nails healthy — minus splits and breaks?

3 Are your nails neatly manicured?

4 Are your knuckles soft and smooth?

5 Are your hands soft and supple on both the outer side and the palms?

Beautiful hands are the result of regular good care. If you find that your hands aren't as pleasing as they should be, the pages that follow will help you dramatically improve their overall appearance.

NAILS

4.

TEN SHINING EXAMPLES OF TIME AND CARE

Hands and nails say a great deal about you to others. You make the difference in what your hands communicate. That is, **care or neglect.** Do your hands deserve compliments or criticisms? When you consider all the hazardous things that can happen to nails, it's not surprising that they're sometimes in less than satisfying shape. But the critical news is this: All you need is a little time on your hands (so to speak) to make a noticeable improvement in their appearance and condition. Read on and discover how you can give your hands and nails lady-of-leisure status.

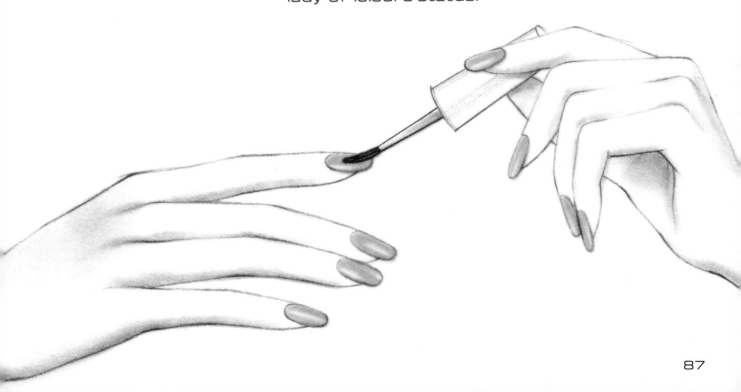

NAILS AND HOW THEY GROW

Here are the facts about the physical structure of your nails that will help you understand the nail's composition and growth pattern.

MATRIX The matrix is the only living part of your nail. Nourished by the bloodstream, the matrix is where nail growth begins.

LUNULA The half-moon or lunula that you see at the base of your nail is the only visible part of the matrix.

CUTICLE The cuticle is the opaque border of skin surrounding your nail. Cuticles should be kept soft and pliable and away from the nail to prevent hangnails.

NAIL PLATE The layer of nail you see is called the nail plate.

FREE EDGE The outer tip of the nail plate that extends past the finger is referred to as the free edge.

FREE EDGE

NAIL PLATE

LUNULA

CUTICLE

MATRIX

POINTERS FOR PROBLEM NAILS

Most nail flaws can be solved rather simply. Listed here are common problems and how to remedy them with the nail products and professional guidance you need.

PROBLEM: SPLIT OR BROKEN NAILS

SOLUTION:

NAIL MENDER KIT In the past, repairing broken nails required the services of a professional manicurist. But now that nail mender kits are available for at-home use, the process is simpler than ever. Follow product directions for salon-perfect results.

PROBLEM: TOO SHORT NAILS OR PROTECTING LONG NAILS

SOLUTION:

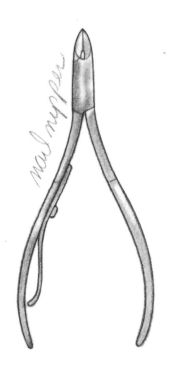

nail nipper

NAIL WRAPPING, once practiced only in beauty salons at prices as high as $50.00, is now available in inexpensive, do-it-yourself kits. Wrapping helps prevent nails from chipping, splitting and peeling.

What's more, it helps prolong the wear of nail enamel. Choose a kit with self-adhesive nail wrap tissues for easy and efficient application. Follow product directions.

LIQUID NAIL WRAP is usually a 2-step treatment that's as easy to apply as nail enamel. There are two liquids to use in the process — one contains nylon fibers that protect the nails from splitting, peeling and breaking, and the other liquid is applied over the first to give nails a smooth, porcelain-like finish.

NAIL HARDENER liquid can be used as a base and/or a top coat. Fortified with nail-hardening ingredients, this liquid protects and hardens weak, soft nails and offers further protection to long ones.

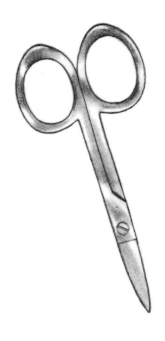

PROBLEM: WEAK OR FRAGILE NAILS

SOLUTION:

NAIL HARDENER
PROTEIN NAIL TREATMENT
LIQUID NAIL WRAP

There are three products that help fortify and strengthen nails — nail hardener, protein nail treatment and liquid nail wrap. All are effective. Read product information and choose the one that is programmed to your needs. You might consider alternating the treatments — nail hardener one week and a protein nail treatment or liquid nail wrap the following week. Weak or fragile nails should be treated continually.

" Nail enamel removers that leave a white, chalky film on nails or cuticles are too drying. Select a gentle remover that makes conditioning claims. If nails are weak or your skin sensitive, select an acetone-free remover. **"**

PROBLEM: WHITE SPOTS OR RIDGES

SOLUTION:

**RIDGE-FILLING LIQUID TREATMENT
NAIL SMOOTHING BOARD
NATURAL NAIL GROWTH**
In time, white spots and ridges will grow out with your nail. Until then, ridges can be cosmetically smoothed over with a special ridge-filling nail product or a special nail smoothing board.

PROBLEM: RAGGED CUTICLES

SOLUTION:

CUTICLE CARE Ragged cuticles and split skin are a result of hardened, overly dry cuticles. Applying cuticle cream regularly and massaging it into cuticles will prevent dryness and cracking. Nightly application is a good idea, as is a weekly treatment with a nail soak. Be sure to apply cuticle remover to eliminate dry, ragged skin. Then gently nudge cuticles back with a manicure stick. Trim with a cuticle nipper or cuticle trimmer only where necessary and after cuticles have been softened with cuticle cream.

PROBLEM: HANGNAILS

SOLUTION:

PROPER NAIL AND CUTICLE CARE As your nail grows, cuticles grow out and will eventually dry up and become rough unless they're kept well lubricated and pushed back from the nail. That's why it's important to use a nail soak and cuticle remover during your weekly manicure, as well as a daily application of cuticle cream.

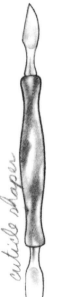

nail whitener pencil

cuticle trimmer

cuticle shaper

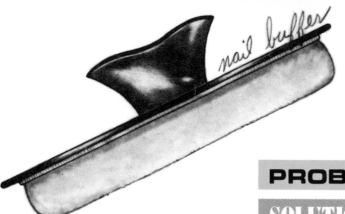

nail buffer

PROBLEM: NAIL BITING

SOLUTION:

STOP Keep an emeryl file with you at all times and use the finer side to eliminate those rough edges that tempt you. Try keeping nails a uniform length (even if they're short) and use nail hardener to protect them against chipping or breaking. If you've acquired the habit of putting your fingers into your mouth, pick up a small object—paper clip, pencil, etc.—and fiddle with it instead. Keeping nails well manicured and polished will also help discourage biting. Remind yourself how lovely your nails will be once you stop stunting their growth.

PROBLEM: NAIL SHAPE

SOLUTION:

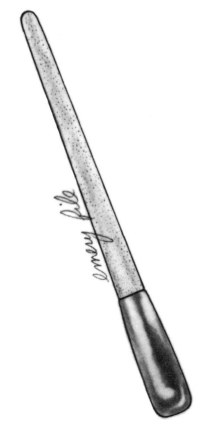

emery file

CUTICLE CARE AND PROPER FILING Carefully pushing back cuticles allows more of your nail to show and consequently appear longer. Use a cuticle massage cream nightly to soften cuticle. Then gently push cuticle back with a manicure stick or a cuticle shaper. Lightly does it, since the lunula is delicate and can be easily damaged. When filing, remember to keep the sides of nails straight and round the corners for a tapered nail shape. Don't file your nails deeply in the corners—allowing them to grow out at the sides provides extra support against breakage. And <u>never</u> "saw" nails back and forth.

PROBLEM: NAIL STAINS

SOLUTION:

BUFFING/BASE COAT Buff your nails as part of your regular manicure. Use a base coat prior to applying nail enamel to help prevent stains from occurring. Another option: Rub fresh lemon across clean nails to gradually fade stains.

PROBLEM: NAIL ENAMEL BUBBLE

SOLUTION:

PROPER APPLICATION Be sure nail surface is properly cleaned with nail enamel remover before applying your base coat and nail enamel. If nail enamel is too thick, use nail enamel solvent for thinning. Resist the temptation to add extra dabs of nail enamel on the first coat — correct mistakes with the second application. Apply enamel away from direct heat or air conditioning vents and allow sufficient drying time between coats. If time doesn't allow for natural drying, use a brush-on or spray nail enamel dryer according to product directions.

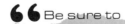

❝ Be sure to wipe off the lip of the nail enamel bottle after each use and keep it tightly capped to avoid premature thickening. ❞

ELEMENTS YOU NEED TO START: Nail enamel remover and cotton balls • emery board or emeryl file • nail soak • cuticle remover • manicure stick or cuticle shaper • cuticle trimmer, scissors or nippers • buffer (optional) • base coat or ridge filler • nail scissors or nail clipper • nail enamel • clear top coat

RECIPE FOR LADY FINGERS

With a little time and the proper nail care tools, you can have nails that pass close inspection...with flying colors.

ONE Start clean. Remove any traces of nail enamel with nail enamel remover.

TWO Begin your nail shape-up. Trim excess nail with nail scissors or nail clip. Then refine shape with an emery board or emeryl file. Gentle, even strokes in one direction from each side of the nail to the center are essential. Refer to NAIL SHAPE on page 92 for more advice.

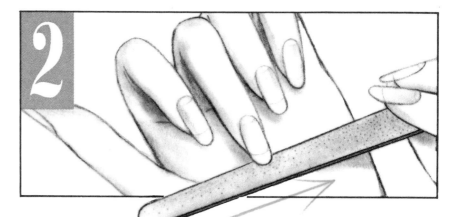

THREE Soak fingers in a nail soak for one minute. As you dry your hands, push back cuticle with a towel.

FOUR Apply cuticle remover around cuticle and under nails. Then gently push back cuticle with a manicure stick or cuticle shaper.

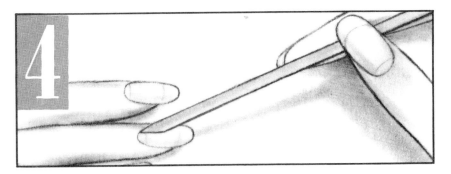

FIVE Clip any excess cuticle or hangnails with cuticle scissors, trimmer or nipper. Cleanse nails in warm, soapy water.

SIX Remove leftover residue with nail enamel remover.

SEVEN Buff nails gently in one direction to bring blood flow to the surface.*

EIGHT Apply base coat to nails. Allow to dry.

NINE Brush on your favorite shade of nail enamel. Use three quick strokes — one down center of the nail and one on each side. Allow 5 minutes, or longer if possible, between coats.

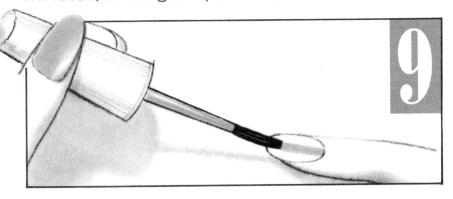

TEN After your enamel is dry (at least 30 minutes) add a top coat or nail hardener. Brush liquid under nail tips for extra protection.

Your salon-perfect manicure should last 7 days. In the meantime, touch up nail tips and chips with added nail enamel and top coat.

*If you do not wish to apply shaded nail enamel, buff nails for natural shine and use a nail whitener pencil under nail tips to highlight natural nail beauty.

1 MANICURE CHECKLIST

If you find your manicure lacks staying power, you may be doing something wrong. Be sure this listing _doesn't_ apply to you.

☐ Nail enamel was too thick. Thin it with nail enamel solvent. Never use nail enamel remover, since it has a negative effect on application and wear.

☐ Nails were not adequately cleaned before nail enamel application. Soaps, oils or other substances may not have been adequately removed from your nail before you applied enamel. So be sure to use remover before you apply base coat.

☐ You didn't allow adequate drying time for your enamel. Apply nail enamel a couple of hours before bedtime or use a liquid or spray-on enamel dryer for quick drying.

☐ You forgot your rubber gloves — detergents, abrasives and scouring pads will chip your polish. Gloves will also help keep the skin on your hands softer, smoother, prettier.

☐ You forgot to apply your top coat under the free edge nail tip for more effective sealing power and longer wear.

☐ You forgot to renew your top coat daily for added protection and extra shine.

NAIL FACTS

A. It takes 4 to 6 months to grow an entirely new nail.

B. The more you massage your cuticles to stimulate the flow of blood and nutrients, the better nails will grow.

C. A diet high in protein is essential to strong, healthy nails.

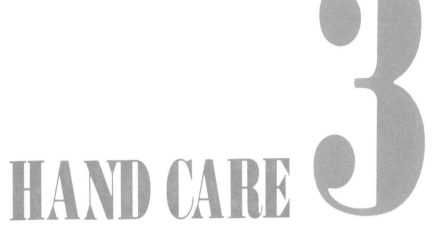

HAND CARE

- Always use a pencil to dial the telephone.

- Pick up small objects with the pads of your fingers.

- Use a medicated lotion on hands that have been overexposed to cold weather or abrasive detergents.

- Smooth on an enriched hand cream before you put on rubber gloves for a beauty treatment while you work.

- Use a pumice stone to gently smooth away callused areas of skin.

- Keep hand lotion on the job, in your purse and in the kitchen and bath to ensure regular use.

Soft, pretty feet demand the same year-round beauty care you devote to your hands and complexion. Keeping your feet in top-notch condition will make them feel good which contributes to your total well-being. With regular foot care, you can avoid problems that make your feet sore or unsightly.

FOOT CARE FOR FLAWLESS FEET

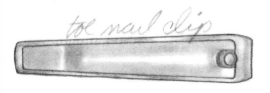

toe nail clip

TREAT YOUR FEET TO A PROFESSIONAL PEDICURE Elements you need to start: nail enamel remover • cotton balls • emery board or emeryl file • nail soak • cuticle remover • manicure stick • toenail clip or toenail nipper • pumice stone or foot groomer • base coat • nail enamel • top coat

FOLLOW THESE SIMPLE STEPS:

- After bath or shower, when feet have been well scrubbed, use a foot groomer or pumice stone to gently smooth calluses and rough skin.

- Remove old nail enamel.

- Trim toenails with toenail clip or toenail nipper in a straight or slightly curved shape. Use an emery board or emeryl file to round the corners of the toenails. Smooth down any rough edges with fine side of your board or file.

- Soak toes in a "nail soak" for a minute or two. As you dry your toes, lightly push back cuticle with towel.

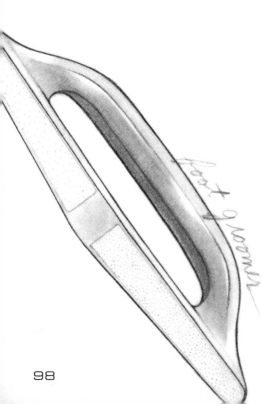

foot groomer

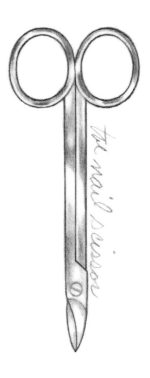

- Apply cuticle remover. Use a manicure stick to gently loosen and remove excess toenail cuticle. Clip excess cuticle with cuticle scissors, nipper or trimmer. Wash toes thoroughly.

- Remove ragged or torn cuticle with cuticle nipper, scissors or trimmer.

- Reapply nail enamel remover to eliminate any excess residue.

- Use a foam rubber separator or weave a tissue in and out between toes.

- Apply base coat.

- Once base coat is dry, apply nail enamel.

- Top coat is optional.

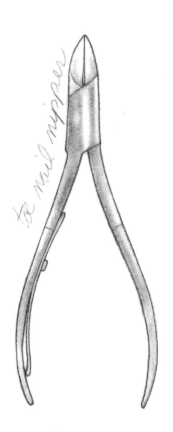

DAILY:

1 Elevate your feet at least 15 minutes each day to help improve circulation.

2 Massage in a rich lotion every night before retiring, concentrating on heels and areas where calluses develop.

3 Refresh hot, tired feet with a scented foot spray or foot powder.

4 Walk barefoot at least 15 minutes each day to give your feet free-form exercise.

5 Alternate the heel heights of your shoes to keep leg and feet muscles well toned.

evaluate your hair

Does it feel brittle
or wiry?
Does it look dull,
unpolished?
Does it act limp
or lazy?
Does it lack bounce
and body?

If you answered "yes" to
even one of these ques-
tions, your hair is not
the best it can be. Hap-
pily, proper care can
change that.

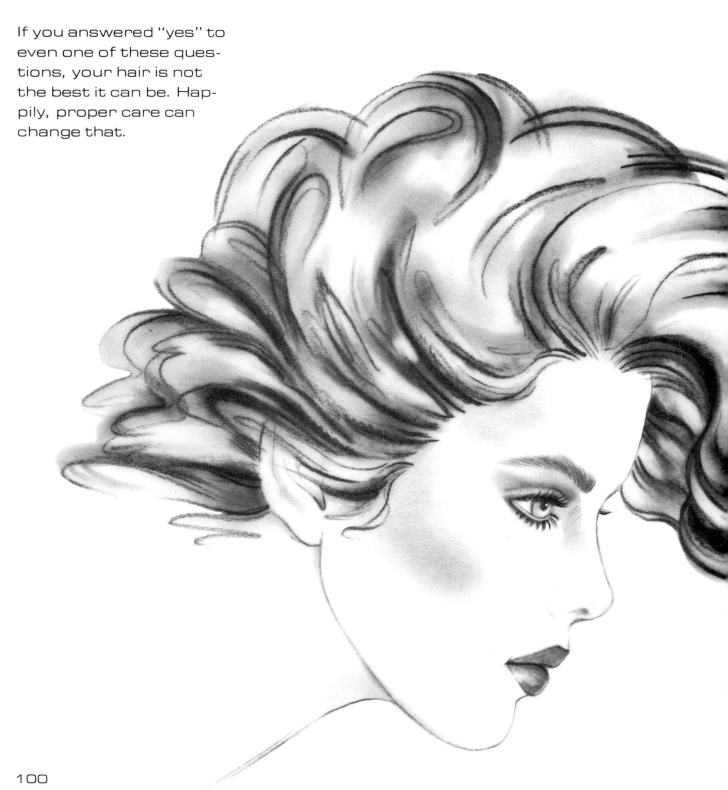

HAIR 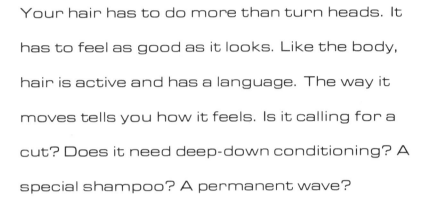 5.

KEEPING IT ALIVE, WELL AND LUSTROUS

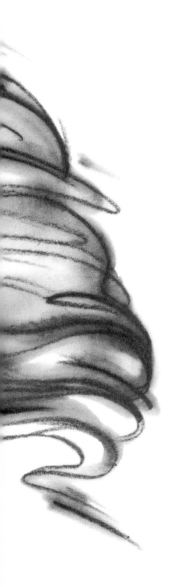

Your hair has to do more than turn heads. It has to feel as good as it looks. Like the body, hair is active and has a language. The way it moves tells you how it feels. Is it calling for a cut? Does it need deep-down conditioning? A special shampoo? A permanent wave?

If you're accustomed to taking shampoos and conditioners off a shelf simply because they're labeled as such, your hair isn't getting what's good for it. Using the right shampoo and conditioner is essential to the way your hair looks, feels and behaves. Hair texture, condition and hair type should be considered.

THE NATURE OF HAIR

To give you a clear and simple understanding of your hair, let's examine it under a microscope. When magnified, a strand of hair shows three layers: cuticle, cortex and medulla.

THE CUTICLE is the protective outer layer of the hair strand. Its hard cells overlap like the tiles on a roof. The condition of hair is principally determined by the cuticle.

THE CORTEX is the second layer and gives hair its color, strength and elasticity. The cortex is where haircolor changes occur during tinting and lightening processes.

THE MEDULLA is the innermost layer of tissue and cells that acts as a supportive structure.

When hair is in healthy condition, the cuticle cells lie flat and reflect light, which gives hair a glossy cast. When hair is damaged, the cuticle becomes rough — absorbs light — and hair looks dull, feels dry and brittle. Before you can accurately determine your hair's needs, you should know the type of hair you have. Essentially, hair falls into three categories:

DRY NORMAL OILY

TEST

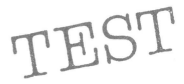

WHAT HAIR TYPE ARE YOU? Take this easy
2-step test to help classify your hair type. First
shampoo your hair. After 24 hours, evaluate its
condition by deciding which of the following 3
descriptions best defines the look and feel of your hair.

DRY

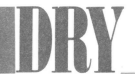

DRY HAIR FEELS BRITTLE AND LOOKS DULL, FRIZZY, ABSENT OF SHINE.

Dry hair is caused by one of two things: A normal result of underactive oil glands or the after-effects of overprocessing with chemicals. When dry hair is unrelated to normal causes, self-help steps are vital.

1 Brush hair daily to help stimulate scalp oils. Twenty or so brushstrokes are adequate. Over-brushing can be harsh on hair.

2 Reduce chemical hair processes, since they can increase dryness and split ends.

3 Shampoo with a product designated for dry or processed hair.

4 Condition your hair after every shampoo.

NORMAL

NORMAL HAIR LOOKS CLEAN, BOUNCY AND SHAMPOO-FRESH.

Because this hair type has no special problems, it is classified as normal. Biologically, normal hair has a balanced oil activity. With proper cleansing and maintenance, normal hair should remain in good and bouncy condition.

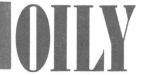OILY

OILY HAIR LOOKS LIMP OR MATTED – ALMOST THE WAY IT APPEARED BEFORE SHAMPOOING.

Oily hair is the result of overactive oil glands. But, at one time or another, even oily hair needs conditioning, since normal things like brushing, rolling, blow-drying and perming can be damaging. What's more, sun, wind and salt water weaken hair and strip it of protective oils. For the best results when conditioning oily hair, apply conditioner to the strands of hair only. Do not apply to the scalp area.

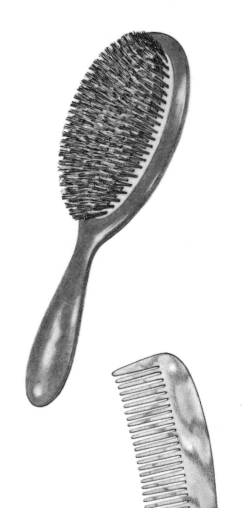

BRUSH-UP

Brushing illuminates the hair by bringing out natural oils. Use a natural-bristled or plastic-bristled brush for gentle care.

There **is** a correct way to brush hair. First, tilt head downward to bring nourishing blood to the scalp. Begin at the hair roots and work in sections, dividing the brushed from the unbrushed. Twenty-five brushstrokes will do it.

While wet hair is easily detangled with a wide-toothed comb, a plastic brush on a cushiony rubber base will also smooth out tangles without unnecessary pulling and tugging.

CHOOSING THE PROPER PRODUCTS

SHAMPOO Your hair attracts dirt from the environment, almost like a filter. The cleansing ingredient in shampoo loosens dirt and oils and partially emulsifies them. In this changed state, hair grime is easily rinsed away.

The shampoo you select should be keyed to your hair type and any special processes—from blow-drying to coloring—that your hair regularly experiences. There are various formulas:

- extra-body formulas for fine hair

- deep-cleansing shampoos for oily hair

- moisturizing shampoos for dry, damaged hair

Shampoos enriched with protein and other beneficial elements give hair an extra boost by helping to fill in cracks and crevices within the cuticle layer. Test shampoos to find the one that does the most for you.

CONDITIONER Conditioners have a natural affinity to the hair for a purely scientific reason—positive and negative attract. Conditioning ingredients are positively charged. When these ingredients are

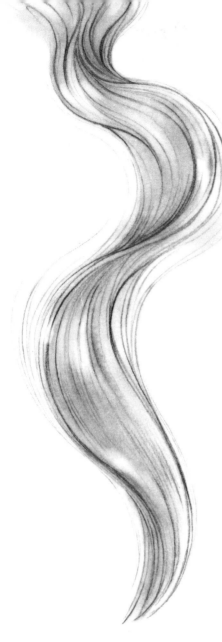

applied to the hair (which is left in a negatively charged state by shampoo), they are attracted to the hair and catch hold of each strand.

THE BENEFITS OF USING A CONDITIONER

- Conditioners are a "life-support system" for hair. They make hair more manageable by eliminating static electricity that causes flyaway hair.

- They help smooth the cuticle surface of hair, which produces glossy shine.

- They help detangle wet hair to reduce damage from pulling and stretching.

Essentially, there are three kinds of conditioners: creme rinses, instant formulas and intensified conditioners. Creme rinses and instant conditioners are time-saving products. Intensified or penetrating formulas are made to remain on the hair for 15 to 30 minutes for the concentrated treatment damaged hair requires.

BASIC STEPS TO DEEP-CONDITIONING

1 Shampoo hair well and rinse.

2 Blot dry with a towel.

3 Section hair; apply conditioner to scalp and hair. Then massage into scalp for 1–2 minutes.

4 Leave on according to product directions. (Heating cap is optional.)

5 Rinse well with warm water.

6 Use a wide-toothed comb to detangle.

BASIC STEPS TO INSTANT CONDITIONING

1. After thoroughly rinsing away shampoo, gently squeeze excess water from hair.

2. Apply sufficient conditioner to cover hair.

3. Allow conditioner to remain on hair for 60 seconds.

4. Rinse thoroughly with warm water until hair feels smooth and tangle-free.

5. Use a wide-toothed comb to lightly smooth away remaining tangles.

Use this Customized Hair Care Guide to Select the Most Efficient Products for Your Hair Type. Remember to Follow Package Direction for Maximum Benefits.

TYPE OF HAIR	CONDITIONER	SHAMPOO	PLUS
BRITTLE, COARSE OR DAMAGED HAIR	Use an intensified conditioner twice a week or after every shampoo. Select a hot oil treatment, a creamy beauty pack or a moisturizing formula. You may also want to alternate these conditioners.	Use an enriched shampoo for dry hair 3 times a week. Protein types are best.	Limit use of blow dryers and heat-styling appliances. Try air-drying instead.
OILY, FINE OR LIMP HAIR	After every other shampooing, use a lightweight conditioner formulated for your hair type to help guard against tangling and give your hair the clean-looking luster it needs. Apply to strands or strand ends, away from your oily scalp.	Shampoo with a deep-cleansing formula or extra-body shampoo.	When dandruff is the result of an oily scalp, use a medicated shampoo every third or fourth shampooing.
NORMAL-TO-DRY HAIR	Apply an instant conditioner each time you shampoo and an intensified formula once a month.	Use a shampoo developed for normal hair or one with built-in conditioners. This combination offers the balanced amount of cleansing and conditioning agents your hair needs.	

THE FAIL-SAFE THEORY: The cut is the basis of any good hairstyle. You should feel comfortable making suggestions to your hair stylist about the look you want. If you find a style you like in a magazine, take the picture along and discuss its possibilities.

FINDING YOUR BEST HAIRSTYLE

A GOOD HAIRCUT should follow the natural flow and fall of your hair to make maintenance easier. Thick, wavy hair, for example, is naturally inclined to a layered hairstyle. If hair is straight and fine, a blunt cut and a permanent wave will give it more thickness, bounce and body.

THE SHAPE, CUT AND STYLE of your hair should enhance your face shape as well. Look at the sketch for your face shape and then in a mirror. Decide if a little rearranging of your hair might lend a better complement to your face.

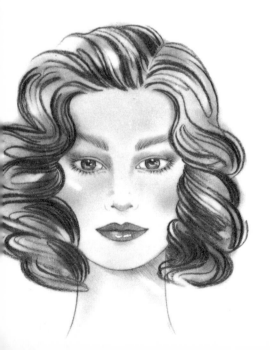

ROUND

Pulling your hair straight back will only emphasize the roundness you are trying to avoid. If your hair is short, wear styles that are fuller at the crown. If your hair is long, it should be worn fuller at the neck to detract from roundness.

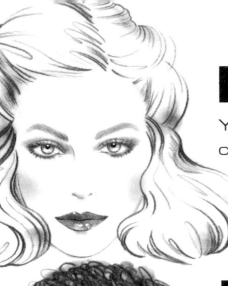

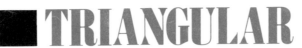 TRIANGULAR

You should wear long, shoulder-bouncing cuts to slim your forehead.

 RECTANGULAR

Bangs that are cut at an angle or styles that are fuller at the sides give the illusion of width.

 SQUARE

A wispy sweep of bangs across the brow will soften your face. Always think softness... curls or waves will take the attention away from your angular edges.

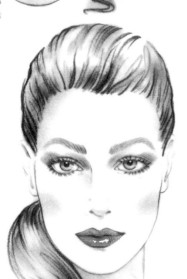

 OVAL

Hairstyles that frame your face are most flattering. Simplicity is key. The styles you choose should not be so fussy that they detract from what nature has already perfected for you.

Haircoloring adds new vibrancy to your hair. Whether you choose a rinse, semi-permanent or permanent coloring, hair color changes should look natural to blend well with skin tone, brows and lashes. Use a deep-conditioner after all haircoloring processes and a shampoo formulated for color-treated hair.

HIGHLIGHTS ON HAIRCOLORING

	DESCRIPTION ▶	RESULTS	REAPPLY
FROSTING KITS	Bleach mixture penetrates the hair shaft and removes natural color by a lightening process.	Dramatically lightens selected strands of hair for a sun-streaked effect.	After 4—6 months, depending on hair length
HAIR-PAINTING KITS	Bleach mixture is painted onto selected strands of hair with a special brush.	Lightens selected top layer strands of hair by 3—4 shades.	After 4—6 months, depending on hair length
METALLIC DYES OR COLOR RESTORERS	Metal-based substances darken grey hair with repeated application.	Produces a deeper tone of grey hair to give a darker overall appearance.	After 4—6 weeks
TWO-STEP BLONDING SYSTEM	Bleach removes natural color from the hair. Toner adds color to hair.	Significantly lightens overall haircolor.	Every 4—6 weeks

	DESCRIPTION ▶		RESULTS	REAPPLY
HENNA		The pulverized leaves and flowers of the Lawsonia inermis plant are called henna. When mixed with water, the henna substance coats the hair.	The orange-red tints warm dark brown and black hair, but the coloring can be too intense on light and grey hair.	After 3—4 months
TEMPORARY LIQUID COLORINGS		Refreshes tinted or toned hair between touch-ups. Tones down "brassiness." Adds color to hair that is faded or sun-bleached. Removes easily with shampoo.	Coats the hair shaft, but does not change natural color.	After each shampoo
			RESULTS	REAPPLY
SEMI-PERMANENT LIQUID COLORINGS		Penetrates the cuticle layer of hair, but does not alter the natural color pigment.	Adds color to grey hair and gives a lift to bland natural color. Will not lighten hair.	After 4—6 shampoos
ONE-STEP PERMANENT LIQUID COLORINGS		Penetrates the hair shaft and changes the natural color pigment. Lightening of the hair pigment occurs as the new haircolor takes hold. Cannot be washed away. Lasts until the hair grows out.	Can dramatically change haircolor to lighter or darker shades. Covers grey completely.	After 4—6 weeks
ONE-STEP GENTLE LIGHTENERS		Penetrates hair shaft to lighten natural haircolor. No color deposit.	Makes hair 1—2 shades lighter.	After 6—8 weeks

Sophisticated

Elegant

Romantic

Sexy

Sensual

FRAGRANCE 6.

PRIVATE PLEASURES FOR THE SENSES

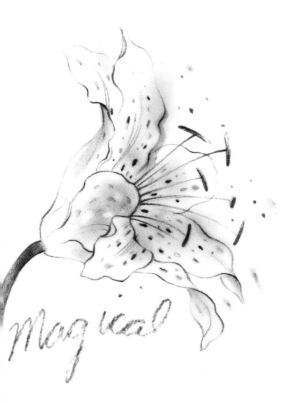

Magical

FRAGRANCE is like love; you can't see it but you know it's there. **Silent and suggestive.** In its infinite mystery and complexity, fragrance influences your feelings and temperament. In a sense, fragrance has the same reflective power as color. Certain scents evoke the **romantic** mood of mauve, others are as **feverish** as fuchsia or as **magical** as gold. Yet every fragrance has one element in common—the element of wonder. Because, mystifyingly, fragrance has the power to entertain your sense of smell.

The scents you select are the **personal signatures** with which you choose to identify yourself, to please yourself and the people around you. What's more, fragrance reveals who you are in purely **sensual** terms. And sensuality is a beautiful fact of a woman's life.

**FRAGRANCE HAS A PROVOCATIVE HIS-
TORY** The art of perfumery literally goes back
to the beginning of time, when aromatic woods
were burned to please the gods. Thus, the
name perfume, which derived from the Latin
words "per fumum," means "through smoke."

HISTORICALLY...

Cavemen and women discovered that the burn-
ing of certain woods caused a soothing feeling
and made the world they lived in more fragrant.

In 800 B.C., the Queen of Sheba admittedly
used the compelling power of perfumes to
entice and seduce King Solomon.

Cleopatra was legendary for scenting the sails
of her barge to command attention during her
passage and to announce her arrival.

When the tomb of King Tutankhamen was
unearthed in 1922 – 3,300 years after his elaborate burial – the aroma of potent fragrances
lingered in the King's ornate perfume bottles.

At resplendent Greek and Roman banquets,
the wings of doves were scented, so that fragrance was emitted as they fluttered about.

The exalted Napoleon Bonaparte, who utilized
over 60 bottles of fragrance each month,
astounded adversaries on the battlefields with
his unexpectedly fragrant presence.

Fragrance can be likened to music, since every scent is composed of a top note, a middle note and a base note. These three components create a chord and perform in concert with one another. Understanding these elements gives special insight into the rare and unusual harmony that fragrance represents.

THE COMPOSITION OF FRAGRANCE

the top note
is the initial scent you receive with the first sniff of a fragrance.

the middle note
is the main body of a fragrance and its principal aromatic theme.

the bottom note
is the lingering aura of the principal aromatic theme of a fragrance.

When one understands that it takes half a ton of rose petals to make one pound of "essential oil of rose," the luxury of fragrance approaches a reality. ONE SCENT MAY HAVE 100 OR MORE DIVERSE ELEMENTS IN ITS DISTINCTIVE BLEND. Once the precious formula for a new fragrance has been determined, the perfume begins to orchestrate each subtle element in the master plan and melds into a final symphonic form.

It is generally agreed by the great perfumers of the world that there are seven basic groups of fragrance to suit your wants and whims. Getting to know the types available will help you develop your own fragrance repertoire.

SINGLE FLORAL: The strength of one flower dominates this essence, even though there are probably pilot notes to augment the main fragrance chord. Single florals can be the scent of gardenia, tea rose, or any fragrant flower.

CATEGORIES OF SCENT

MODERN FLORAL BLEND: As the name suggests, florals are almost literally a nosegay of wonderfully compatible flowers that blend to complement each other. They also contain a complex combination of synthetic scents.

GREEN: As gloriously fresh and outdoorsy as a wooded glade, this fragrance type is a distinctive combination of herbs, ferns and oakmoss.

SPICY: Think of a fragrant soufflé of scent that includes cinnamon, ginger, cloves, vanilla and carnation. The resultant fragrance is long-lasting, haunting and nostalgic.

CITRUS BLENDS: An effervescent fragrance type that conjures up a happy mood. Lively accents of lemon, mandarin, lime and other citrus elements create this blend.

ORIENTAL BLENDS: Sultry, exotic — a blended tapestry of opulence and warmth. Some blends fuse sandalwood with patchouli and musk.

FOREST BLEND: A classically sophisticated fragrance blend accented with qualities of oakmoss and amber. Floral, fruity or fresh green notes impart interesting subtlety.

SELECTING A SCENT

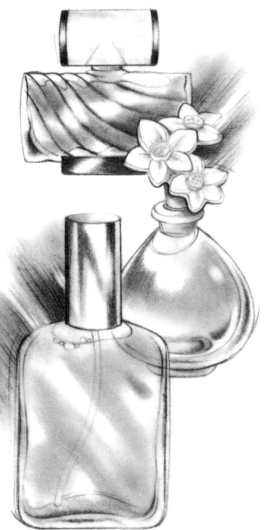

TO TEST the true essence of a fragrance, it's important to allow the scent to develop on your skin. Apply fragrance on the pulse point at the inside of your wrist. Wait 10 minutes to be certain you evaluate the middle note or main body of the fragrance before you make your choice.

FRAGRANCE is not unlike a kaleidoscope — offering many views and lights and dimensions. It can be highly spirited or tenderly romantic. A scent can conjure up silky fields of cool grass or take a different aromatic avenue and impart to the wearer an aura of sophistication or a sense of fantasy.

PUT SOME PLANNING into your search for new fragrances. Experimenting takes time and testing too many scents at once will defeat your goal to find the fragrances that are right for you. Make your selections with the same time and care you devote to other investments and treasures.

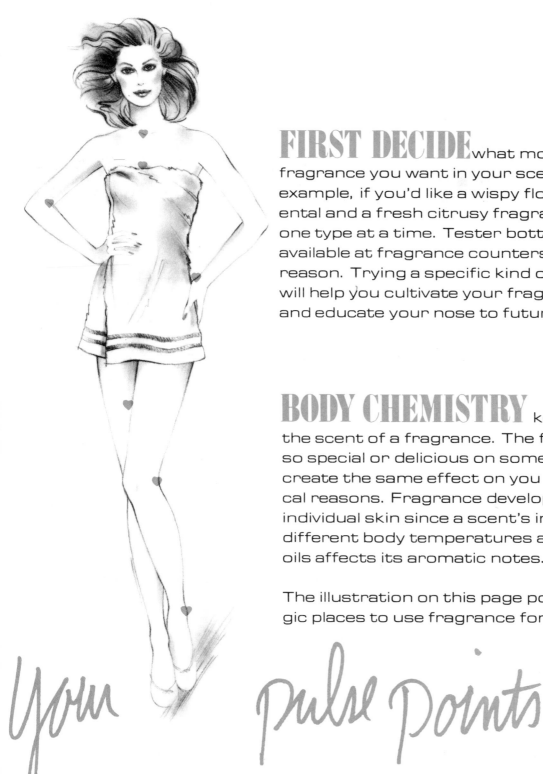

FIRST DECIDE what moods or kinds of fragrance you want in your scent collection. For example, if you'd like a wispy floral, an exotic oriental and a fresh citrusy fragrance, shop for one type at a time. Tester bottles are always available at fragrance counters for just that reason. Trying a specific kind of scent at a time will help you cultivate your fragrance knowledge and educate your nose to future selections.

BODY CHEMISTRY keenly influences the scent of a fragrance. The fragrance that is so special or delicious on someone else may not create the same effect on you for purely biological reasons. Fragrance develops differently on individual skin since a scent's interaction with different body temperatures and natural skin oils affects its aromatic notes.

The illustration on this page points out strategic places to use fragrance for sensual effect.

Your pulse points

One fragrance can be translated into different forms and each has its own depth and wearing power. Within these various categories of scent are sprays, pours, portables, touch-tips and solid forms for every need and moment throughout the day.

THE FAMILY OF FRAGRANCE

PERFUME is the longest-lasting and most intense form of scent, since it contains the highest percentage of perfume oil. Apply it to pulse points and allow your body to transmit its fragrant message. On and on and on.

CONCENTRATED COLOGNE OR EAU DE TOILETTE are second in perfume intensity. Because the composition of the fragrance is suspended in an alcohol base, they are an ideal all-over body refresher.

COLOGNE is the most delicate and subtle form of fragrance. It is never heavy or overpowering and the length of its lasting aura depends on individual body chemistry.

SPLASH OR EAU FRAICHE are refreshing, wispy fragrance forms with a subtle toning quality. Lighter than cologne, they are designed to be used lavishly and have a delightful effect after the bath.

PROTECT THE POWER OF SCENTS

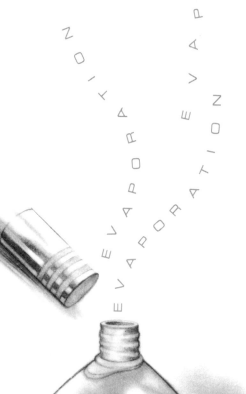

EVEVAPORAPORATION EVAPORATION EVAPORATION

Perfume is as fleeting as it is rare. It longs to dance out of the bottle to mingle with the air. Once the bottle is opened, it has a tendency to evaporate. So bottle stoppers must be anchored with a decided twist to maintain a perfume's life and true character.

Perfume pales under heat and sun, so to keep your fragrances at peak potency keep them in a cool, dark, dry place or refrigerate them.

When you've received a large bottle of fragrance, think about transferring it into smaller containers, so that the fragrance can be carried in your purse, a bottle kept in your office, and so on. Separate fragrance into the various bottles you wish to use with an eyedropper or small funnel.

Perfume demands that you use it, so make it a delicious treat in your daily beauty ritual.

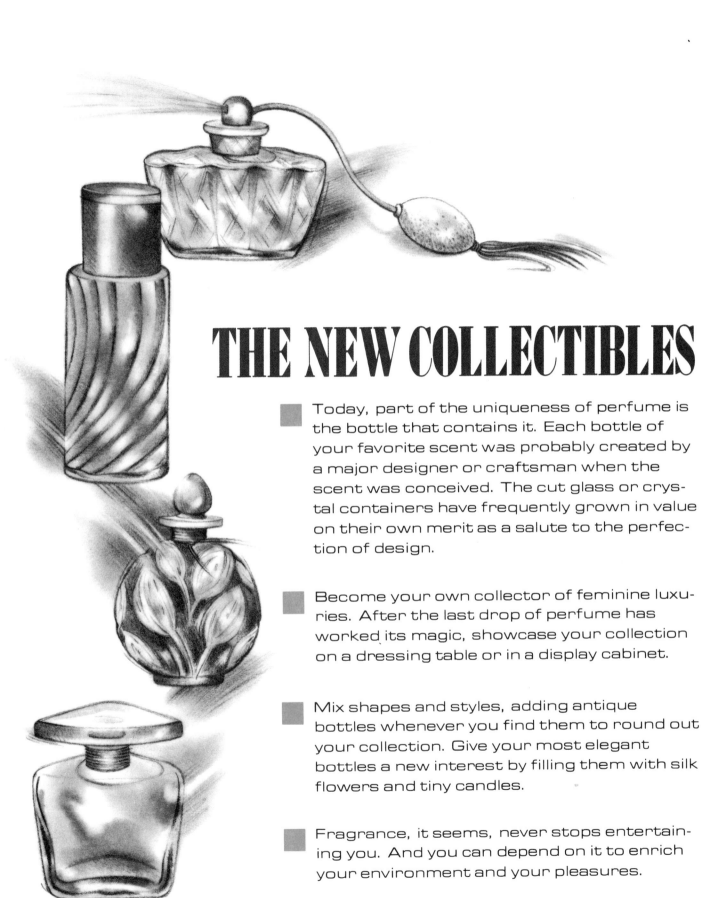

THE NEW COLLECTIBLES

Today, part of the uniqueness of perfume is the bottle that contains it. Each bottle of your favorite scent was probably created by a major designer or craftsman when the scent was conceived. The cut glass or crystal containers have frequently grown in value on their own merit as a salute to the perfection of design.

Become your own collector of feminine luxuries. After the last drop of perfume has worked its magic, showcase your collection on a dressing table or in a display cabinet.

Mix shapes and styles, adding antique bottles whenever you find them to round out your collection. Give your most elegant bottles a new interest by filling them with silk flowers and tiny candles.

Fragrance, it seems, never stops entertaining you. And you can depend on it to enrich your environment and your pleasures.

Entering a house with a pleasing air is a profound pleasure. Fragrance enlivens an environment as it reflects individual taste and style. Just as there are many moods of scents for you to wear, fragrance can evoke an array of atmospheres in your home. Let your imagination keep you on the scent of originality.

AROMATIC MOODS AT HOME

LIVING ROOM Keep fragrant candles on a table or mantel. ● Spritz air-conditioner with fragrance before guests arrive.

BEDROOM Place scented soaps or sachets in lingerie drawer. ● Spritz sheets and pillowcases with a romantically scented fragrance. (Spray a corner of sheet to be sure fragrance doesn't stain.) ● Hang a bone china pomander ball on bedposts. ● Spray silk or dried flowers with a single floral fragrance.

DINING AREA Make a table bouquet with jonquil, freesia, roses or other fragrant flowers.

BATH Scent bath and hand towels with a citrus fragrance. ● Keep potpourri and a basket of scented soaps on display.

KITCHEN Hang an orange pomander near the stove to catch rising heat. ● Rub oranges and lemons with citrus oil and arrange in a basket. ● Fill a brandy snifter with cinnamon sticks and cloves. ● Make a spice potpourri with mint, sage, basil and rosemary.

HALL CLOSET Spray padded clothes hangers with fragrance. ● Line shelves with scented shelf paper. ● Place pomanders or sachets strategically.

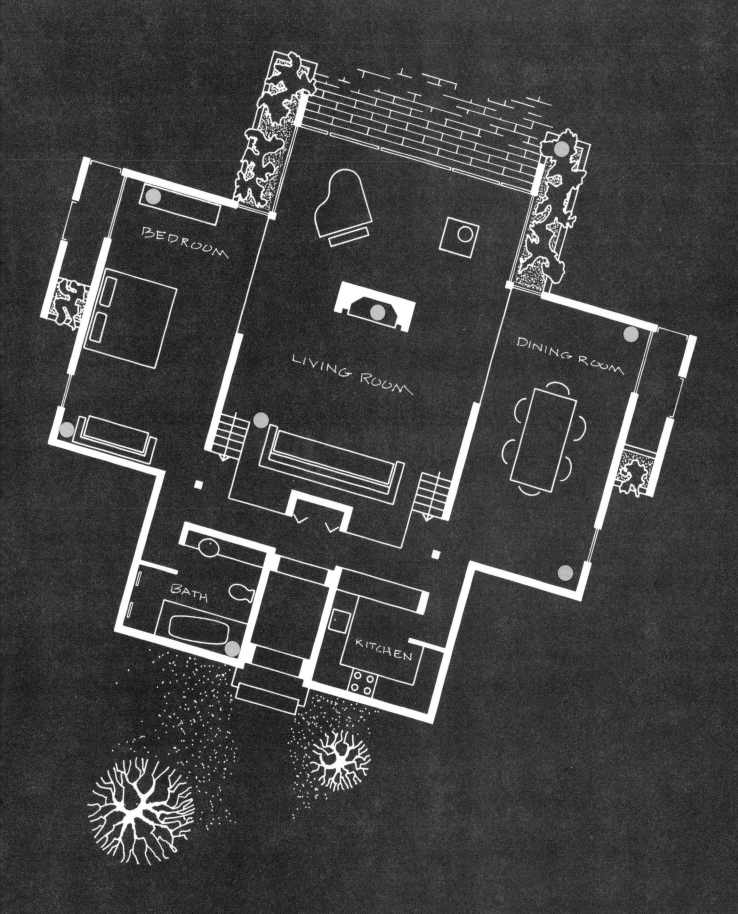

This floor plan offers suggestions for vivid ways
to use fragrance throughout your living space.

The bath is much more than a way to keep your body fresh and clean — it's a great escape to a private world. Indulge yourself in the one retreat where you can close the door, break away from the stress of the day, and bask in that delicious feeling of being cared for.

BATH AND BODY PLEASURES

Whether you want to rev up or relax, you merit more than a warm tub and bar of soap. A leisurely bath is an affordable luxury and, with a bit of orchestration, a bath can turn into a fantasy of fragrances and an oasis of pleasure. And the more self-prescribed pleasure you impart to your life, the better you feel. And the healthier you look.

BATH PRODUCTS

The array of fragrant bath and body products is growing wider and richer. And they're all designed to treat your body gently and lavishly. Because whether you pause to realize it or not, your body is a natural wonder and is entitled to all the rewards of its status.

The priceless value of bath products lies in the fact that they stimulate an active interest in body care. Enriched with the air of fragrance, these products not only help tone and condition your body, but impart a silky scent to your skin.

SCENTED SOAPS should be fundamental to your bathing ritual. Many of these soaps contain encapsulated moisturizers that release in water for gentle, all-over moisturizing and leave the skin silky soft.

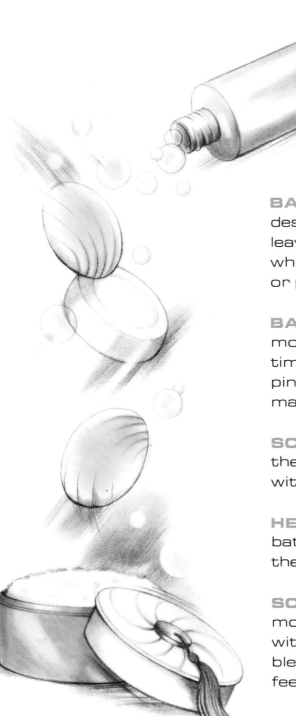

BATH GELS are gentle body cleansers designed to be used in place of soap bars. They leave a delicate aura of fragrance on the skin which can be heightened by layering on cologne or perfume from the same fragrance family.

BATH OILS added to the water give skin the moisture and lubricants that harsh weather or time may have taken away. Use care when stepping in and out of the bath, since bath oil can make the tub surface somewhat slippery.

SCENTED BATH CRYSTALS are fun, since they fill the air with fragrance and enliven water with mood-provoking color.

HERBAL BATH BEADS impart the feeling of bathing in a wooded glen and your body reaps the benefits of nature's own loving care.

SCENTED BUBBLE BATH creates a magical mood. There's wonderful whimsy in bubbles with their small outbursts of scent. Most bubble baths contain emollients that make your skin feel satin-soft.

MILK BATH softens the skin and leaves it silky. Select one in your favorite scent and invest in its companion, scented soap, for a total experience.

THE BATH DOESN'T STOP HERE ANYMORE
After the bath, lightly towel dry so skin is left slightly damp. Follow with a fragrant body lotion applied with massaging strokes. In winter weather, consider applying a scented bath oil for its extra lubricating effects. Finish with a cloud of fragrant dusting powder and cologne or perfume. When layering fragrance, remember to use the various fragrance forms in the same scent for a lasting impression.

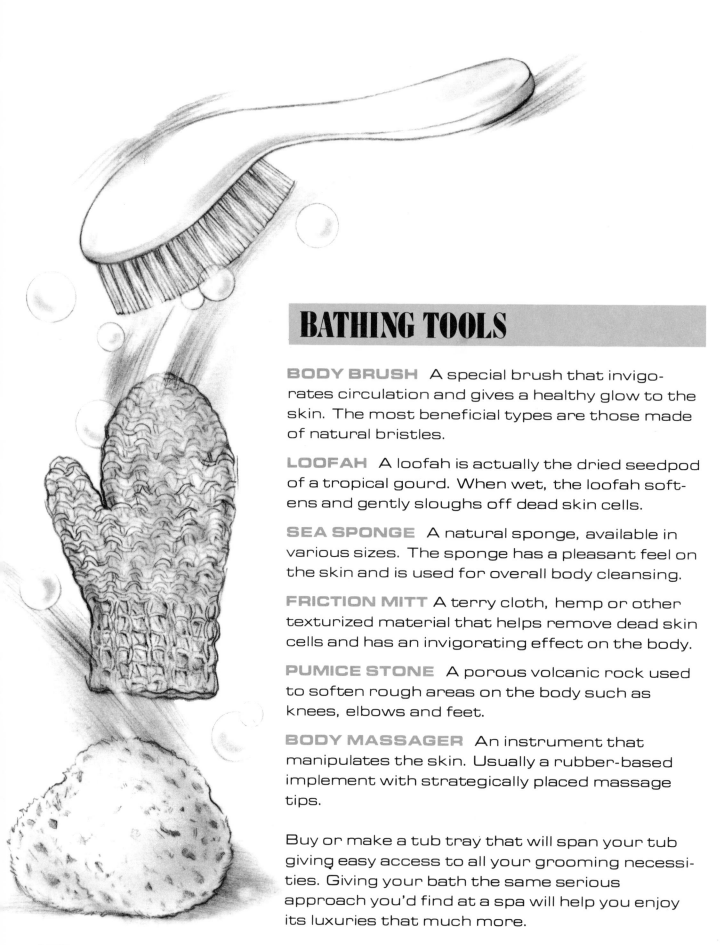

BATHING TOOLS

BODY BRUSH A special brush that invigorates circulation and gives a healthy glow to the skin. The most beneficial types are those made of natural bristles.

LOOFAH A loofah is actually the dried seedpod of a tropical gourd. When wet, the loofah softens and gently sloughs off dead skin cells.

SEA SPONGE A natural sponge, available in various sizes. The sponge has a pleasant feel on the skin and is used for overall body cleansing.

FRICTION MITT A terry cloth, hemp or other texturized material that helps remove dead skin cells and has an invigorating effect on the body.

PUMICE STONE A porous volcanic rock used to soften rough areas on the body such as knees, elbows and feet.

BODY MASSAGER An instrument that manipulates the skin. Usually a rubber-based implement with strategically placed massage tips.

Buy or make a tub tray that will span your tub giving easy access to all your grooming necessities. Giving your bath the same serious approach you'd find at a spa will help you enjoy its luxuries that much more.

THE BATH AS A BEAUTYOASIS

Water temperature is the difference between relaxing and reviving. According to hydro-therapy experts, the best bath or shower temperature is 98° to 100°F. In other words, the ideal bath water is approximately the same as your natural body temperature. But the great thing about a bath is the many moods it can create and the various ways in which it can alter your state.

the invigorating bath

THE ENERGIZING ELEMENTS: fragrant bath gel or soap, a glass of effervescent mineral water, a loofah or friction mitt and a body brush. Step into a warm bath. Then let out half of the water and add a flow of cool water to allow your body a gradual cool down to the water temperature. Lather your loofah or friction mitt with bath gel for its energizing effect. Scrub back and shoulders with body brush and, before stepping out, drink the mineral water as a final pick-me-up.

the soothing bath

THE LULLING ELEMENTS: perfumed bath oil, bath crystals, fluffy bath towel, facecloth, herbal eye pads. Draw a warm bath, keeping temperature between 98° and 100°F for ultimate relaxation. Add perfumed bath oil and bath crystals for their soft color and scent. Be certain to use bath products as your tub is filling so that they thoroughly disperse into water and the bouquet permeates the air. Once you're in the bath, roll bath towel into a neck rest, place herbal pads on your eyes and let your thoughts drift for half an hour while the fragrance and bath oil work their magic on your psyche and body.

the fantasy bath

THE MAGICAL ELEMENTS: candles, spray fragrance, fresh flower petals, a refreshing beverage, soft music, scented soap, bubble bath. Draw a warm bath and add your favorite bubble bath product. Spray flower petals with fragrance and sprinkle them in bath water. Light candles and place around tub and face basin. With your beverage nearby and music set at a soothing tone, step into the candle-glowing water and reflect on beautiful things.

in addition ▶

ABOUT THE AUTHOR

Revlon has been making women beautiful for five colorful decades. The year it all began was 1932. The founder: Charles Revson. The place: New York, New York.

America was in the depths of the Depression. Luxury was a forgotten word as the once wealthy now sold apples in the cold. Women looked unfinished. Plain. Almost no one, save ladies of the theatre, enhanced their natural attributes with cosmetics.

REVLON felt the moment had come to change the face of the world and bring new enrichment to millions of women. The Company's plan was to make a true nail enamel, a dress for the nails that could be made in any color. And if it could be made in any color, why not make it in the more individualistic colors than the light, medium and dark shades of the times?

WITH THIS CHALLENGE in mind, Revlon created nail enamels in a series of vibrant pinks and reds... colors totally changed from anything womankind had ever seen.

NEW AVENUES of beauty emerged as Revlon initiated a fashion breakthrough: matching lips and fingertips. This innovative concept was reflected in the names created by Revlon for the new coordinated shades.

NAMES LIKE Fire and Ice, Raven Red, Cherries in the Snow, Million Dollar Red mirrored a thrilling connection between the way a woman felt and the image she presented to the world.

FEMALE RESPONSES were changing— and Revlon was changing them. The Company introduced the first cream eyeshadow, the first all-in-one makeups, the first waterproof base mascara, the first blush-on and the first fashionable lipstick cartridge.

THESE DEVELOPMENTS prompted Revlon to institute a dynamic research program. Exhaustive study resulted in new product forms like hypoallergenic/fragrance-free cosmetics and special beauty treatments for delicate skin.

AS BUSINESS GREW, and as other companies began to make cosmetic products, Revlon continued to remain the undisputed leader. It was leadership forged out of Revlon's conviction that women deserved products which would help them develop their fullest beauty potential.

THUS, REVLON progressed from a small team of men in the early thirties to a bountiful corporation whose success is dependent upon the efforts and ideas of approximately 37,000 people in 130 countries throughout the world.

To many people, cosmetics and fragrances appear to spring from the imagination. But the art of a beauty product is founded upon disciplined, well-reasoned scientific knowledge. To produce results with that knowledge is the business of the Revlon Research Center—one of the most advanced cosmetic laboratories in the world.

THE SCIENCE OF REVLON COSMETICS

The Revlon Research Center represents the technical, developmental and quality control arm of Revlon in all its worldwide operations.

The Center provides technical support and new product development for the various markets around the world. Primary activity involves the translation of formulas and processes and revised methods of manufacturing.

The creation of a new skin care cream, blush, body or face lotion, lipstick, nail enamel or fragrance comprises a trial, literally, by fire and ice. The trial employs ultrasophisticated, automated, analytical instrumentation, as well as microscopes, test tubes, computers, climatic chambers, heating and cooling to extremes, and volunteer testing. Ultimately, the product and package are put in a test oven where they remain for weeks at 120° Fahrenheit.

Just as a prime goal of putting a man on the Moon was getting him safely back to Earth, the prime mission of the Research Center's work is not only enhancing the quality of life, but also doing it with surety that is universally reliable.

The Center's 150 scientists and technicians work in a score of laboratories that accommodate the individualized testing required for makeup, creams and lotions, lipstick, nail enamel, toiletries, haircolor and hair preparations, and fragrances. Formulas are developed according to their specialties and tested for behavior and quality of use.

Among the many product development probes for safety and integrity, a microbiology lab works with the formula to make certain that the product is clean and stays clean during its reasonable lifetime. Pharmacologists and toxicologists assault the product with the same battery of safety test procedures used for the development of a pharmaceutical. But not until innumerable use-testing on both men and women establishes performance as well as safety is the formula approved for marketing.

Thus, it is only after many months, even years, of meticulous testing that a beauty product makes intimate contact with the consumer.

All these activities may start from dreams that sound plucked from the Arabian Nights — jasmine, patchouli and sandalwood. They may spring from a law of nature or a chance discovery. But before they appear on the marketplace and then on you in wondrous color and scent, they have traveled painstakingly through the clean white rooms where technicians and scientists work.

1932 1942 1952 1962

1972   1982

1982 marks Revlon's 50th Anniversary. The Company's colorful past and present have helped women create images of drama, emotion and beauty. It is an accomplishment that society celebrates, for woman gives mood and motion to beauty. Her needs, dreams and desires have yielded priceless ingredients in the creation of color and cosmetics.

Thus, Revlon and woman have formed an inseparable association. With certainty, the years to come hold promise of still newer explorations into the fine art of beauty.

1992   2002

Warmest Wishes for a life of Beauty

REVLON